Henry A. Hartt

The Columbian Institute:

For the preservation of health and the cure of chronic diseases

Henry A. Hartt

The Columbian Institute:
For the preservation of health and the cure of chronic diseases

ISBN/EAN: 9783337731359

Printed in Europe, USA, Canada, Australia, Japan

Cover: Foto ©ninafisch / pixelio.de

More available books at **www.hansebooks.com**

THE COLUMBIAN INSTITUTE;

FOR THE

PRESERVATION OF HEALTH

AND THE

CURE OF CHRONIC DISEASES.

By HENRY A. HARTT, M. D.

NEW YORK:
RUSSELL BROTHERS, PRINTERS, 17, 19, 21, 23 ROSE STREET.
1878.

PREFACE.

This book, as far as its great object is concerned, speaks for itself. A preface is required only to forestall the criticisms which the new enterprise, to which it relates, must inevitably encounter. The late distinguished surgeon and noble hearted man, Dr. Krackowizer, whose loss the whole profession in this city deplores, said to me, in the presence of his colleague, a few weeks before his death: "The institution which you propose is much needed, and I am satisfied that you are laboring to establish it for the benefit of science and humanity, but everybody does not know you as well as I do, and you must prepare to meet with unjust suspicion and reproach." I was then engaged in the effort to obtain the indorsement of the Medical Faculty of New York, my success in which demonstrated their power to act with justice, manliness, and virtual unanimity on a great question of public and professional interest. It cannot be denied, however, that the originator of any important undertaking is obliged to pursue a course which renders him liable to various charges, the first of which, generally, is that of egotism. Now, there is no man who feels greater repugnance to self-laudation than myself, or to that which is next akin to it—the publication of encomiums bestowed by the kindness and gratitude of those to whom valuable services have been rendered by him. On this account I did not present to the public meeting a number of letters sent to me in behalf of the institution by patients who, in the warmth of their feelings, gave glowing descriptions of the results of my treatment. I would, indeed, have been glad if I could have safely and properly excluded from the proceedings thereof everything in the shape of personal praise. But it must be remembered that I am endeavoring to procure from the people a large sum of money, not to provide a home for incurables, nor a theatre for experimentation, but to found a hospital for diseases that are generally regarded as incurable, yet which, I maintain, on the basis of facts obtained in a professional career of more than forty years, can be radically and permanently cured.

I am naturally inclined to expect that, when I testify to that which I have seen and know, my word will be accepted; but from long intercourse with the world I have discovered that, in dealing with subjects with reference to which a marked and wide spread incredulity exists, no one can afford to dispense entirely with the testimony of others.

I do not conceal my methods or my remedies. I use only agencies that are purely scientific and open to all; and I make no pretension to powers that do not belong to other medical men, if they choose to exercise them. In my paper on the Prevention and Curability of Chronic Diseases, I have clearly indicated the general principles that govern me in their management, and some of the principal means that I rely upon for their cure; and, as soon as practicable, I intend, according to my intimation therein, to publish my opinions and practice in detail with regard to several diseases of a chronic nature that are exceedingly prevalent, and that are wrongly considered incurable.

In the prosecution of the work that I have taken in hand, I desire to act in full concert with my brethren, my aim and purpose being to benefit mankind and to promote the highest interests of my profession.

HENRY A. HARTT, M. D.,

142 *East Thirty-fourth Street,* N. Y.

CONTENTS.

CHAPTER I.
The Prevention and Curability of Chronic Diseases........... 5

CHAPTER II.
Indorsement by the Faculty................................ 37

CHAPTER III.
Indorsement by the Citizens............................... 50

CHAPTER IV.
Proceedings of the Committee.............................. 76

CHAPTER V.
Plan for the Establishment of the Institute............... 105

CHAPTER VI.
Necessity for the Institute............................... 108

THE COLUMBIAN INSTITUTE.

CHAPTER I.

I read a paper before the New York Medical Library and Journal Association some time ago, which, on account of its relation to the proposed institution, is here reproduced.

THE PREVENTION AND CURABILITY OF CHRONIC DISEASES.

I have been requested by several eminent physicians of New York to give to the profession and the world the general results of my observation and experience during the forty-two years that I have been engaged in the study and practice of medicine.

I was educated in Scotland, at the University of Glasgow, in what may properly be styled the heroic school, wherein I was taught that the lancet was to the physician what the sword was to the warrior. In those days the chambers of the sick were scenes of combat, in which blood flowed almost as freely as upon the battle field. The great ruling idea was the necessity of depletion. It was demanded for every ailment and for every accident, and the fear that haunted the mind of the conscientious practitioner, in almost every case, was that he had neglected to take away a sufficient quantity of blood. When the veins had yielded up the last drop it was safe to abstract. then followed counter-irritation in its harshest forms, by means of the fly-blister, the tartar emetic ointment, Granville's lotion, the issue by caustic potassa, and by nitric acid, the seton, the moxa, and the actual cautery. To these were superadded, in many cases, a succession of drastic purgatives and hydragogue cathartics. As soon as the powers of the system were sufficiently reduced, the aid of mercury was invoked. The strongest preparations of the medicine were preferred, and it was generally considered necessary to push it to the extent of producing salivation, which was regarded as the only evidence that it had affected the system. It cannot be denied that these measures were generally effectual in subduing inflammatory affections in their most formidable aspects, but it is equally certain that they sometimes also destroyed the patient. I do not remember any case in my own practice in which they proved positively fatal, but I can recall an instance in which a man was carried by the use of the lancet so near to the gates of death that an indelible impression was made upon my mind, and ever since I have exercised more caution in its employment. The patient lived at the distance of twenty-five miles from my residence, and I was obliged to travel by night, through a burned forest, in the most terrific thunderstorm I ever saw. I reached my destination at two o'clock in the morning, and found that the patient had been suffering for several days from a severe attack of pneumonia. The length of time it had existed, and the ravages it had committed on the powers of the system, suggested a doubt with regard to the propriety of depletion. But I had never seen nor heard of an instance of recovery from this disease without it, much less had I been informed that it has a natural tendency to a cure, and having no leeches or cupping apparatus at hand, I opened a vein in the arm, but when I had obtained about half a pint of blood the patient fell back in a faint, from which he rallied slowly, and then only to gasp and pant for hours as though his end had come, in spite of the most powerful stimulants. He had not fully recovered from this condition when I was obliged to leave him, and thirty hours elapsed before I could see him again. I shall never forget the anxiety I felt on his account during that period. I found him, however, decidedly convalescent.

There may have been a time in which the stamina of mankind demanded and bore this rigorous treatment. But that era had passed, and it was no longer required. The strain had become too great. A reaction was inevitable, and it came, and like reactions generally, *it has gone entirely too far.* The pendulum has swung to the other side. It has been powerfully aided by a remarkable change which has taken place in the type of disease. It is impossible to deny that acute diseases do not now make their appearance in the same violent form that they did thirty or forty years ago. An inflammation or fever which was then attended with a pulse of from one hundred and twenty to one hundred and sixty, full and bounding, gives us now a much softer pulse of from ninety-six to one hundred and eight, with all the other symptoms correspondingly mild. I have obtained the testimony of many distinguished physicians, in both this city and elsewhere, and all agree with me upon this point. It may be difficult to ascertain the causes of this variation in the character of acute diseases, but the fact remains.

The reaction in question received also a great momentum from the changes produced in the constitutions of men by the progress of our civilization. As nations advance in commerce and the arts, they acquire habits of ease and luxury, and lose in proportion their moral and physical force. Their powers of endurance are weakened, and there is a general revolt against everything that is painful, disagreeable, or unpalatable. They would take from fire the property of giving pain, though every child that should be born thereafter should run the risk of being burned to death, and they would extract from every medicine its nauseous taste, though every man might be poisoned by using it as an article of food. They lose sight of the great fact that, in both the moral and the physical departments of nature, the violation of law is followed by punishment, and that all remedial measures are necessarily disciplinary, and, therefore, distasteful; and so they demand of their spiritual advisers that they should prophesy smooth things, and cry "peace, peace," when there is no peace, and of their medical advisers that they should treat them only with rose water, and lemonade. In perfect harmony with this new spirit of luxury and folly came homœopathy, holding in its hand a vial of sugar pellets, and proposing to thrust aside at one fell swoop the accumulated results of the wisdom and experience of ages, and proclaiming the law of *similia similibus curantur* as the one great and only law of medical science. If the multitudes who embraced this heresy had paused to examine the subject, they would have seen at once that it is never by such sudden and revolutionary measures that any science or art is advanced; that, on the contrary, it is by the gradual addition of new discoveries of fact and principle and law that the great structure is slowly reared from age to age, never to be completed till time shall end. They would have seen, also, that that which has been so ostentatiously put forth as the only law of medical science is simply a law which applies to certain classes of agents called stimulants and tonics. From time immemorial it has been known that if these agents are used in excess they produce a weakness of the parts upon which they operate, and that if these parts have become debilitated or congested, through cold, or an injury, or any other cause, then these agents, in moderate doses, are the appropriate remedies. They would have seen, also, in pursuing the inquiry, that there are other agents of vast importance which act upon the law of opposites, and others again which act upon principles different from either. In short, they would have discovered that the laws which govern the action of medicines are varied and manifold, and that the attempt to restrict the science of medicine to one law is just as ridiculous as the pretence that all the ills that flesh is heir to can be cured by one remedy. And, if they had chosen to go still further, and examine into the *practice of the founder* of the system, they would have met with facts which would have both amused and astounded them. For instance, in his work entitled the "Organon," he says: "In a sudden affection of the stomach, with frequent nauseous eructations, as of spoiled food, accompanied with depression of mind, cold at the feet, hands, etc., if the patient should only smell once a globule of sugar the size of a mustard seed, impregnated with the thirtieth dilution of pulsatilla, then he is cured in the space of two hours." Now, Professor Simpson, of Edinburgh, in his admirable work upon homœopathy, has shown that this thirtieth dilution of pulsatilla, according to the prescribed formula, is one grain of pulsatilla dissolved in an ocean of alcohol equal to several globes, the diameter of which would reach from this earth to the nearest fixed star. If Hahnemann had declared that he was the Emperor of Germany, or the King of the Cannibal Islands, he would not have made a statement a whit more preposterous or incredible. And yet, in a later work, he affirms, as the result of his matured experience, that a dose of the two hundredth dilution is the best dose for all diseases, both acute and chronic!

And now I come to the inquiry, what have the Faculty done to withstand homœopathy and resist the spirit of the age? Have they studied and weighed the modification which has occurred in the type of disease, and carefully adjusted their methods to meet that modification? Have they manfully stood up for the dignity of the science, purged it of its errors, and under its venerable banners, in the name of God and humanity, despised the blandishments of fashion, rebuked the effeminacy of the times, and insisted upon a vigorous and effective system of treatment? It is not my province to prefer a charge against my brethren, or to impugn their motives, but I am bound to declare my solemn conviction that the practice of medicine, at the present day, is sadly deficient in force and vigor, and that if it continues much longer in its downward course, it will become as weak and powerless as homœopathy itself. This imbecility has already begun to produce its legitimate fruits. I have reason to believe that there are men of eminence in the profession, distinguished for their knowledge of pathology and skill in diagnosis, who, when they come to the great object of their art, confess their want of confidence in the power of medicine to cure disease. The young men come forth from the laboratory and lecture-room with their minds fully stored with every kind of technicality and lore; but, when they are called upon to grapple with the terrible realities of professional life, they hesitate and know not what course to pursue.

The imbecility of modern practice is most strikingly shown in the *prevalence of chronic diseases, and in the general scepticism, both in the profession and out of it, with regard to their curability.* The first point, I believe, is universally admitted, and requires no argument. If there were any doubt on the subject I think it would be dispelled by the fact, which was mentioned to me by a friend who visited Wies Baden last summer, that there were at least twenty-five thousand persons there who had come to avail themselves of the remedial power of the waters. With respect to the general disbelief in the curability of chronic diseases, I think it can easily be established beyond dispute. There are special institutions for certain classes of chronic disease, but, as far as I know, there is not in the world a hospital for the treatment and cure of chronic diseases generally.

It would be a most unjust and unwarrantable reflection upon the Christian benevolence of mankind to suppose that the sufferers from these terrible maladies would be left thus unprovided for, if it were not generally conceded that they could not be cured. And what means the almost universal practice on the part of physicians of ordering them off to different parts of the world for change of air—a policy which was at one time confined to the rich, but which now is often extended most ridiculously to the poor, who have not a penny to carry them away? I cannot but regard it as a most humiliating confession of the impotency of their art. The utter hopelessness into which the patients themselves ultimately fall is another proof of the discouragements they meet with on every side. A man will not readily accept the idea that he is the victim of a life-long disease. He goes from place to place, consulting physicians, charlatans, and clairvoyants, and using nostrums of every description, and grasping convulsively at every straw that is thrown out to him, till finally he resigns himself to his fate, and the voice of an angel itself could not awaken within him a spark of hope. In some severe cases the mind becomes a wreck, and the man loses all moral power, and can no longer make the slightest effort for his own deliverance. One of the saddest spectacles I ever saw was that of a poor fellow who was lying in a basement, on a miserable cot, to which he had been bound by the chains of rheumatism for seven years. At night he could not sleep, but tossed about, as far as his stiffened and painful limbs would permit, in perpetual agony. By day he slept a little, and felt no pain except on motion, and then he cried aloud. I pitied him and offered to treat him gratuitously, but he promptly and positively declined, saying, "Greenwood is my only refuge and hope." I saw an old man recently whose lower limbs have been greatly weakened by the action of the rheumatic poison on his spinal cord, so that for two years he has scarcely been able to walk, even with crutches. He has become utterly indifferent to every earthly object, himself included. I asked him if he would be willing that I should treat him if he were sure that I could cure him at once, so that he would be able to throw away his crutches and walk about the next day as well as he ever did. "Why," said he, "that would be a miracle." "Would you allow me to perform that miracle upon you?" "Well, I don't know. I'm not sure that I would."

In order to satisfy myself more fully upon the subject in question, I have made inquiries of physicians and others. I asked Dr. B——, chief of the medical staff of one of our most prominent and useful institutions, what his opinion was with regard to the curability of chronic diseases. He replied: "The fact that they are chronic shows that they are not very curable." A few years ago I inquired of a medical officer of the department of charities and correction the number of patients that were admitted every month with chronic rheumatism, chronic bronchitis, and asthma. He told me that, on an average, they received thirty with rheumatism, twenty-four with bronchitis, and from twelve to twenty-four with asthma. I then asked him, "How many with rheumatism are cured?" He replied, "None." "How many with bronchitis?" "None." "How many with asthma?" "None." "What then," I said, "do you do with these unfortunate patients?" "We relieve them, and the first fine day we discharge them, and take care not to receive them back again if we can avoid it." The resident physician of one of our largest hospitals informed me that the officers of that institution would not receive cases of chronic disease at all. I inquired the reason, and he replied: "First, we cannot be sure of curing one of them; secondly, we cannot hope in the most favorable circumstances to cure more than eight per cent.; and thirdly, it would take very long to restore even that limited number." I asked a physician of great ability, who had been in good practice for several years, what he thought were the chances of cure in the most favorable cases of chronic disease. His reply was, "A happy possibility." A gentleman recently consulted Dr. B——, a prominent physician of Brooklyn, with reference to a relative who had suffered from rheumatism for many years. He said that he would not undertake to treat the case, for he could not cure it, if he were to obtain a fee of fifty thousand dollars. He added that the best thing the patient could do would be to go where there was no rheumatism. Alas for the fate of the sufferers from rheumatism! Asthmatics and others may find a refuge in some favored regions on this globe, but they who are afflicted with this disease must henceforth be remanded to some other sphere. This advice reminds me of an anecdote told me by a friend of mine who has never married, and who, like bachelors in general, has a morbid tendency to scrutinize all his sensations, and who has not, therefore, for many years been entirely free from pain. He met one day a clergyman of his acquaintance, and, in reply to the usual salutation, remarked that he felt very well with the exception of a pain in his back. "Ah," said the sympathizing pastor, "that is very distressing, but it is a comfort to think that when you reach that house not made with hands, eternal in the heavens, you will have no more pain in your back."

I called one day upon my friend Dr. R——, one of the ablest surgeons in this city, to request him to visit with me the child of Mrs. T——, who had been accidentally shot in the head by his brother. I found the doctor just recovering from an attack of rheumatic gout, which had continued ten weeks. He had been subject to the disease, at intervals, for many years. I inquired how much of the time during the ten weeks he had suffered severe pain. He replied: "I suffered agony for four weeks." I said, "Why do you not allow me to cure you?" "Cure me! that is impossible; I have tried everything." "You are going to see a child with me to-day," I said, "whose mother is a living witness to the fallacy of your opinion." After our consultation upon the case of the child, he questioned Mrs. T—— with regard to herself. She told him that she had suffered from rheumatic gout in its worst form for five years, and had been perfectly cured for an equal length of time. "Have you had no return of the disease whatever?" "None." "You were fortunate," he said, "to fall into the hands of Dr. Hartt." But although the doctor has had the opportunity to enjoy a similar good fortune, he has thus far declined to avail himself of it.

The following extract, a minor editorial of the *Tribune*, is, I think, as appropriate as it is amusing:

"Apropos of rheumatism. John Trotman, of Wathena, Mo., was a great sufferer from this incorrigible infirmity. Physicians were in vain, and were likely to be, inasmuch as the complaint was rheumatism, and the patient was sixty years old. So Mr. Trotman, in the absence of his wife, tied two flat irons under his chin and (in some unaccountable way) his hands behind his back, and thus accoutred plunged into Peter's Creek, where he was found soon after quite free from rheumatism and from everything else except the flat irons. The man who was hired to watch Mr. Trotman, and who didn't watch him, hasn't been arrested, though he should be, and at least fined for mitigated manslaughter. The kind of rheumatism which they have in Connecticut doesn't seem to affect the mind, but it is very steady and lasting. A doctor was called in East Hartford to a man, aged sixty-six, who was excessively rheumatical. 'How long have you had it?' says the doctor. 'Forty years,' responded the sufferer. The doctor left without prescribing. We cannot tell how much we should like to see even a partial list of the remedies to which during his life our Connecticut martyr has probably resorted. He has carried a roll of brimstone in his left pantaloons pocket; he has carried a bit of magnetized iron in his right ditto; he has floated, so to speak, in pain killer; he has put his trust in 'cam-fire,' and likewise in capsicum. Whatsoever things are hot or bracing, or tonic or rubefacient, he has resorted to; to the 'king of pain,' to the 'ready and rapturous relief,' to oils, to ointments, to poor man's porous plasters, to red flannel shirts, to galvanic braces, to opodeldoc, to herbs and roots and seeds—to all things which grow or flow, which are digged from the bowels of the earth, which are extorted from crucibles, which drop from retorts, which are rosy or pale in apothecaries' bottles; to powders, to tinctures, to decoctions, to pills, to essences, to panaceas, and to elixirs; to boluses and globules and infinitesimal dilutions; to hot rum and water; to cold gin and sugar; to brandy plain; to sweats and to starvation; to flesh diet, and to fish diet, and to fowl diet—and all in vain."

An article appeared in the London *Lancet* in September, 1869, by Dr. Elam, entitled, "Medicine, Disease and Death," the object of which was to show that from the year 1838 to the year 1868 there had been a decline in the art of medicine. It was based on statistics derived from the annual reports of the registrar general, from which it appeared that the death rate during the period above mentioned had increased about one in a thousand, which corresponded to 3,000 additional deaths in London alone, and to about 22,000 in the whole of England and Wales. It is not necessary to my argument to institute such a comparison, for I have admitted that grave errors existed in the practice of medicine at the time when the alleged retrogression began; but if the conclusion at which the author has arrived be correct, it demonstrates that excessive vigor is not so bad as excessive weakness. In this, as in other things, "to be weak is miserable." The nature of the profession demands strength—strength in the practitioner and strength in his art. It brings a man in perpetual contact with the sorrows and infirmities of human nature. He bears on his shoulders day and night the tremendous responsibility of life and health. The dearest interests and most sacred secrets of society are committed to his care. The lovely infant, the prattling child, the blooming virgin, the ambitious youth, the idolized mother with all her blushing honors thick upon her, the strong man in his prime, and the hoary head of age, all, in their hour of trial and agony, come to him, and depend upon his wisdom and skill. What has he to do with fashion, or prejudice, or taste? Firm as a rock, yet gentle as a dove, he must resist every influence that would turn him aside from the path of duty, and carry out with inflexible integrity the inexorable laws of science. With philosophic candor and sense, in the spirit of the mighty Paul, he should "prove all things, and hold fast that which is good." He should, of course, be willing to make a reasonable trial of new measures or remedies, but the results of experience he should never surrender. And as the physician should be strong, so should there be strength in his art. Although the man that was born blind did not sin, nor his parents, still the great army of sufferers who have contracted their diseases after their birth, must receive, I fear, a harsher judgment. At any rate, they are amenable to the charge of having violated physical laws, and we know that to those laws is invariably affixed a rigorous penalty. The great declaration, that the way of transgressors is hard, applies in this life with almost equal force to violators of law in every department, and it is not more certain that through sorrow and pain and self-denial the spiritual wanderer must go back to the regions of purity and love, than that, by a similar road, the pilgrim of disease must find again the priceless gems of health and happiness. I wonder it has never struck the advocates of expectancy and sugar pellets that nature has given to almost all medicines a nauseous taste, and to many of them a disagreeable odor; and that if the *vis medicatrix naturæ* is as effective and reliable as they imagine, the existence of such a vast array of remedial appliances in the world is a grand superfluity and waste. No; disease is a positive thing, arising from the violation of law, and all analogy teaches us that its treatment must be both positive and painful. It is in vain to attempt to escape the decree. On the one side is Scylla, on the other Charybdis—*pain or death.*

I have said that within the last forty years a change has taken place in the type of disease, and I firmly believe that if medical men throughout the world had modified their treatment so as to make it correspond thereto, and had availed themselves of all the facilities which the march of science has put at their command, neither homœopathy nor any other phase of quackery could have obtained a foothold. But, unfortunately, some of the most important and effective measures—measures which had stood the test of centuries, were almost, if not entirely abandoned. Is it possible that our fathers were altogether mistaken with regard to the principle of depletion in cases of inflammation and congestion? They undoubtedly carried it too far in many instances, but was it not founded on a rational theory, and when practised in moderation was it not attended with the happiest results? It was originally suggested, I doubt not, by the spontaneous hemorrhages which so often occur in congestive diseases, and by the sudden and marvellous relief which they afford. I myself can bear witness to the magical effect produced both by general and local bleeding in numberless instances of acute disease. The abstraction of blood from the arm diminishes the force of the circulation, reduces the temperature of the body, and prepares the way for the more effectual administration of internal remedies. In pneumonia, in pleurisy, in peritonitis, in apoplexy, in puerperal convulsions, in inflammation of the brain, and in active congestions generally, I have seen it produce immediate and striking alleviation of the most alarming symptoms. Formerly, when the lancet was almost universally employed in cases of apoplexy, the general rule was that the patient did not die till the third attack. The man is fortunate now who survives the first. Before the doctrine was taught that pneumonia has a natural tendency to a cure, it was treated both by general and local bleeding, followed by liberal doses of tartar emetic. I doubt very much whether Laennec or his followers ever had to record the terrible mortality from that disease which we have witnessed in these later years; and I can affirm most solemnly that I have treated it with almost uniform success. I was summoned not long ago, at the suggestion of a Catholic priest, who had been sent for to administer the last rites of the church, in the case of a man who had a severe congestion of the upper lobe of the right lung, and who had been treated with stimulants and left to die. It was too late for general bleeding; I therefore applied a dozen leeches over the part affected, and gave small doses of *potassæ et antimonii tartras*, and in twenty-four hours his respiration and pulse were reduced to the natural standard, and in a week he was entirely cured. Local depletion in this manner subdues the force of the circulation and diminishes the quantity of blood in the congested part. I am persuaded that the Faculty have made a grave mistake in renouncing to so great an extent the practice of blood letting, and I trust it will not be long before they will resume it in a moderate and rational degree. The removal of a pint or three half pints of blood from the arm in the beginning of an acute inflammation, immediately succeeded by appropriate internal remedies, will often cut it short in twenty-four or forty-eight hours, whereas, with less vigorous treatment, it would probably continue for several weeks, and possibly assume a chronic character.

The concession to the popular prejudice against mercury is one of the most lamentable features of the time. If there ever was a remedy for which the whole human race should be devoutly thankful it is this despised and persecuted drug. It has been made the object of the bitterest satire and ridicule, and thousands who have died for want of it have left the world with most mistaken feelings of enmity in their hearts against it. Like depletion, its priceless value led to its abuse. It constitutes an infallible antidote, *when properly administered*, to one of the most terrible diseases that vice has entailed upon humanity, and acts specifically as a stimulant upon one of the most important organs of the human system. The attempt to substitute in its place iodide of potassium in the one case, and bismuth and podophyllin in the other, would furnish a fit subject for merriment if it had not been attended with such mournful consequences. The appalling prevalence of syphilis to-day, and the acknowledged incompetency of modern practice to control it, and the frightful mortality among children from diseases of the chylopoetic viscera, I attribute to this unfortunate departure from the ancient landmarks. The error committed in former times with reference to this medicine was its indiscriminate employment in almost all conceivable diseases as an alterative, and to the extent of producing salivation, under the impression that this result was required as an evidence that it had produced its legitimate effect upon the system, and upon the particular affection for which it was administered. In my view of the subject, salivation is a provision of nature to guard against the excessive use of the drug, a sort of lighthouse to warn us from the rocks upon which we might otherwise run—an object which we should always steer away from and carefully avoid. In a future paper, which I propose to publish on the subject of syphilis, I shall give my views at length on the use of mercury in that disease, and I will add at present only, that I deem it invaluable as a remedy for congestion of the liver, and of the intestinal canal, for the purpose of purgation, in combination with other laxatives, and to promote the action of the absorbents in various cases of recent deposit and effusion.

The most remarkable change, perhaps, that has taken place in the practice of medicine is the general disuse of counter-irritation. From the moxa and the actual cautery we have come down to the mustard leaf and ginger poultices. And yet, I confidently affirm, as the result of my observation, that there is *no medicine in the world for internal administration* which exerts one twentieth part of the power of counter-irritants over chronic inflammation. The bougie is not more necessary for a stricture of the urethra, nor are stimulating applications to an inflamed eye or throat or uterus, than these powerful agents are to those internal congestions which cannot be reached by the probe or the syringe. It is strange, that since we have ascertained the law of reflex action, by which alone their chief *modus operandi* can be scientifically explained, we have consigned them to the limbo of the past, thus recklessly setting aside, at one and the same time, the results of experience and the light of modern discovery. We know that a stimulant applied to the extremities of the nerves on the surface of any portion of the body, is conveyed to the cerebro-spinal and ganglionic centres, and thence, by the law above referred to, is transmitted to all the internal ramifications of the complicated net work to which they belong. We have thus, fortunately, the power of acting upon those deep seated congestions which are inaccessible to the eye and the hand, and if we wisely follow the analogy and pursue the same principles of treatment which govern us in those that are external, our efforts will be crowned with similar success. In the case of an external congestion of a chronic nature, it is occasionally requisite to use a powerful caustic; but, as a rule, the application of stimulants is sufficient to overcome the disease. In like manner, an internal congestion of long standing may sometimes demand a seton or a moxa, but generally a milder counter-irritant will answer every purpose. In both cases, however, *it is absolutely necessary that the stimulating application should be repeated at short intervals and for a length of time.* As far as this proposition applies to external congestions, it will be accepted as a matter of course. An oculist, for instance, who should propose to cure a patient with granular lids by touching them once a month with a ten grain solution of the nitrate of silver, or by making a similar application every second day for two or three times, or who, failing in his object after such preposterous experiments, should throw up his case in despair, would justly be laughed at by his brethren throughout the world. But it is not a whit less ridiculous to attempt to master an obstinate bronchitis or spinal congestion by the employment of a mild counter-irritant once a month, or two or three times at shorter intervals, or failing therein, to abandon the disease as hopeless.

There is a second principle upon which counter-irritants act which gives them a decided advantage over mere stimulants. By a law of the animal economy, the existence of a sore on any part of the body causes the force of the circulation to be directed thither. Counter-irritants, by virtue of this law, determine the blood to the surface, and so relieve internal capillaries in a state of congestion of their burden.

The learned and able secretary of the Medical Library and Journal Association, Dr. Andrew H. Smith, has, I think, conclusively shown, in a paper published in the *New York Medical Journal*, for April, 1872, that this effect is still further increased by the rapidity with which the blood flows through the vessels of the irritated part.

He says: "The question is not how much blood the vessels of the irritated part will hold, but how much they will transmit in a given time. This will become evident when we consider that a given amount of blood passes through the capillaries of the body in each unit of time, and is transferred from the arterial to the venous side of the circulation, and that the quantity passing through any one part must affect that passing through the remainder of the body, since the latter must be the exact complement of the former. Thus, if in a given time four pounds of blood pass through the capillaries of the entire body, and one pound passes through the capillaries of the arms, it follows that three pounds must pass through the remainder of the capillary system. Now, if we plunge the arms into hot water and dilate the vessels so that an additional half pound passes through them, the remaining vessels will transmit only two and one half pounds, and the tissues which they supply will be deprived for the time of one sixth of their nourishment. It will be perceived that this is a matter entirely apart from the quantity of blood which might be contained in the arms if severed from the body. The consideration of the increase in the carrying power of tubes, in comparison with the increase in their diameter, involves some of the most interesting points in the mechanics of fluids. The resistance to the passage of the fluid being derived chiefly from the friction against the sides of the tube, will increase in proportion to the ratio of the circumference to the area of the section. Now, the circumference of a circle increases directly as the diameter, while the area increases as the square of the diameter. The friction is obtained by dividing the circumference by the area, and therefore decreases directly as the diameter increases, as is shown by the following formula:

Diam.	Circum.	Area.	Friction.	
a	b	c	$\dfrac{b}{c}$	
$2a$	$2b$	$4c$	$\dfrac{2b}{4c}$	$= \dfrac{b}{2c}$

"From which it appears that doubling the diameter of a tube quadruples its area, and at the same time divides the friction by two. But, great as is this disparity, it is immensely increased in practice, especially when the tube is of very small calibre, and tortuous or branching. The following experiments serve to show how slight an increase in the diameter of a tube will suffice to augment its carrying power enormously:

"Experiment I. A caoutchouc tube of five m. m. bore and three feet long, perfectly straight and of uniform diameter, was found to transmit a given quantity of water in one hundred and fifteen seconds. Another tube of six m. m. diameter, but perfectly similar in other respects, transmitted the same quantity in sixty-five seconds. In this case an increase in the diameter of twenty per cent., and in the area of less than forty per cent., gives an increase in the carrying power of nearly one hundred per cent.

"Experiment II. A glass tube ten inches in length and having an inside diameter of .052 inch, gave passage to six drachms of water in one hundred and twenty-two seconds. Another tube of the same length and under the same condition, but having a diameter of .08 inch, transmitted the same quantity of water in twenty seconds. In this case the addition of one half to the diameter of the tube allowed the passage of six times the quantity of fluid.

"Experiment III. The same tubes were used as in the last experiment, and all the conditions were the same, except that defibrinated bullock's blood was employed instead of water. The blood was previously strained through very fine linen. The smaller tube required one thousand four hundred and forty seconds to transmit six drachms, while the larger tube gave passage to the same quantity in one hundred and forty-two seconds. The ratio here is one half to ten, instead of one half to six, as when water was employed.

"In applying the results obtained from these experiments to the question of counter irritation, we find that certain stimuli applied to the skin act in such a way upon the vaso-motor nerves as to cause a relaxation of the terminal arteries and a dilatation of the capillaries. If the irritation be considerable, the surface assumes a bright scarlet hue in the place of its previous flesh color. Such a change in the color implies a very considerable increase in the diameter of the capillaries."

A memorable case of our own times affords such a striking illustration of the value of counter-irritation, that I deem it appropriate to refer to it in the discussion of this subject. In the spring of 1856, Charles Sumner was struck down in the Senate chamber, by Preston S. Brooks, and beaten on the head with a cane till he became insensible. He was sitting at his desk when the attack was made upon him, and in his efforts to free himself from the hands of his assailant, he sprained his spine in two places. Some time after the assault, I read in a newspaper a letter written by a lady, containing a particular account of his symptoms, from which I inferred that the spine was the seat of disease. In the summer of 1857, I mentioned my opinion to the Rev. Dr. George B. Cheever, and Mr Palmer Waters, of Salem, Mass., who, learning, soon afterward, that Mr. Sumner was lodging at the Brevoort House, in this city, called upon me to request that I would visit him in company with them, and state to him the views which I had formed of his case. I opened the conversation by asking him whether he had any reason to suppose that his spine was affected. He replied, "I am sure it is not, for my physicians examined my spine only yesterday, and assured me that it was perfectly sound." I did not deem it proper, whether rightly or wrongly, to make any further remark to him on the subject, but when we withdrew, I said to the gentlemen who accompanied me, "Nevertheless, his spine is the seat of disease, and no cure can be accomplished until it is properly treated." At our interview, he informed us that he had consulted several eminent physicians, both in this country and in Europe, and that all had agreed that he was suffering from an affection of the brain. He said, with tears in his eyes, "I am not afraid to die, but I confess that I do shrink with dread from the thought of insanity."

A month or two afterward he went to Paris and placed himself under the care of Dr. Brown-Séquard, who discovered that the spine and cervical sympathetic were seriously affected, and who treated him successfully by counter-irritation in its severest form. There was everything about this case which was calculated to produce the most profound impression upon mankind. The character and position of the sufferer, the cause for which he was assailed, the boldness and savageness of the attack, the insatiable malice of his enemies which pursued him with misrepresentations, and charged him, in the midst of his agonies, with the ineffable meanness of feigning to be ill, in order that he might extort a sympathy which he did not deserve, all conspired to awaken an unparalleled interest throughout the civilized world. The details of the treatment were published at the time with the utmost particularity, and everybody knew exactly the method by which the cure was effected, and the great physician, who was known before as an ingenious experimentalist and learned physiologist, at once obtained a world wide celebrity as a practical man on account of this astonishing achievement. One would have thought that counter-irritation might now have successfully asserted its claims and become, at least, the fashion of the hour, but the great forces that rule the world were too strong for it, and the horrors of the moxa outweighed the brilliancy of the cure. I would not take one leaf from the crown of Dr. Brown-Séquard, for he is entitled to immortal fame and to the ceaseless gratitude of the American people and of mankind for the energy, fidelity, persistence, and skill which he displayed in the treatment of the wisest and purest statesman which this country has produced; but, I feel that it is my duty, in the interest of science, to declare my opinion that a milder counter-irritant, which would have admitted of frequent application, which would not have been attended with one tenth part of the pain, and which would have been wholly unaccompanied with the prostrating shock of the moxa, would have been equally efficacious in overcoming the disease.

The element of water is one of the most wonderful objects of contemplation. In its various forms of ocean, river, lake, brook, cataract, ice, snow, vapor, and dew, it contributes to the gratification and welfare of man. It constitutes, at one time, the grandest, at another, the most beautiful feature of natural scenery. It supplies the great highways of commerce, and drives its ponderous vehicles with the force of the whirlwind. It holds in its vast bosom and nourishes an innumerable multitude of living creatures, many of which are used as articles of luxury, while many more disport themselves in its mysterious caverns and never have anything to do with the ways or wants or habitations of mankind. Along with its great coadjutors, light and heat, it fructifies the earth and causes it to bring forth plant, and flower, and grain, and fruit, in their season. It is the source of purification throughout the world, and an essential part of the food of man and beast and every living thing. And, in addition to all this vast array of uses and benefits, it is a potent and valuable medicine. If used in combination with ice, or in the form of ice, it serves as a refrigerant, diminishing heat and action, and restoring the tone of weakened capillaries. If employed by means of what is called a "pack," or in the manner of the vapor bath, it becomes a most powerful diaphoretic, driving the blood to the surface, and exciting the exhalants into active operation, so as to remove a large portion of serum and, along therewith, a quantity of any morbid matter that may happen to be in the system. I have known several instances in which the vapor bath has exerted an almost magical influence in the commencement of bronchial pneumonia. The first patient upon whom I tried it was my own son, when he was about four years of age. The disease attacked him in a violent form. His pulse rose to more than one hundred and sixty, and his respiration to seventy-two. In six hours the force of the inflammation was subdued. I adopted this practice upon my own responsibility. There was a time when the warm bath was prescribed for the convulsions and colics of children, and vapor was used to break up a cold or a fever; but latterly, I believe, this treatment has been generally abandoned, and, with the exception of ice, the whole agency of water is given over into the hands of the proprietors of water cure and mineral water establishments. These gentlemen, I understand, for the most part are totally unlearned in medical science, and generally begin their course by informing their patients that they are saturated with drugs, that their diseases in a great measure arise from that cause, and that the first step towards recovery is an entire abstinence from all internal medication. In some simple cases of chronic congestion, the subjects of which have considerable stamina, they may undoubtedly effect a cure. But when the congestion is connected with great debility, or is complicated with some poison in the blood, which cannot be eradicated without internal remedies, they may produce irreparable mischief. A married lady, thirty years of age, who was affected with rheumatism at the age of twenty, and was afterward subject to it for eight years, having two attacks every spring, each lasting six weeks, and generally one in the autumn, applied to me for treatment. She had been attended by homœopathists without benefit, but had been assured by them that if she lived to be more than thirty years of age she would get over it. She grew weary of her burden before the time appointed arrived, and had recourse to an establishment in this city, where she was treated with water exclusively in different ways. By this means the poison was driven from the fibrous tissues, and it afterwards attacked the left lung. She coughed constantly for more than two years before she came to me, when her lung, both anteriorly and posteriorly, was studded with softened tubercles.

There is an institution in this city which proposes, I believe, to cure every description of chronic disease by means of rubbing and passive motion. The system is called the Swedish movement cure; but I doubt if Sweden ever saw one tenth of the curious inventions which are thus ascribed to her. There is every kind of mechanism driven by steam to fulfil the objects designed, and if the molecular theory of our modern scientists be true, and heat and light and life and everything be only a mode of motion, then the pretensions of this establishment, comprehensive as they are, may not prove to be so extravagant as at first sight they appear. But, as I prefer to be governed by the fundamental principle of the Baconian philosophy, which requires an adequate basis of facts before an attempt is made to construct a theory, and cannot, therefore, with Prof. Tyndall, carry my vision beyond all experimental evidence to see anything, much less to behold in matter "the promise and potency of every form and quality of life," I decidedly demur to the proposition that any change of atoms or molecules produced by rubbing and passive motion will cure the various kinds of chronic disease. At the same time, I do believe that this treatment is admirably adapted to promote absorption and restore the tone of parts that are weak from long disuse or otherwise, or that are partially paralyzed, and that if it were used in such cases, in conjunction with electricity or galvanism, it would often be attended with the most satisfactory results.

But why should this or any other important agency be allowed to remain exclusively in the hands of ignorant pretenders, or of those who, though enlightened, put themselves on a level with that class by restricting themselves to a single method of treatment; for it has ever seemed to me that in this partial practice, more than anything else, consists the essence of charlatanism? I suggest the expediency of establishing an institution in this city, under the superintendence and control of the Faculty, with every facility for the use of electricity, galvanism, water in every shape, rubbing and passive motion, to which private practitioners may send their patients, with the perfect assurance that they will receive the treatment prescribed in the best manner, at a reasonable cost, and without being tampered with. I trust that no objection will be made to the employment of any of these important remedies on the ground that the stain of quackery is upon them, either because they have been monopolized, in a great measure, by pretenders or irregular practitioners, or because some of the methods by which they are most effectually applied have originated with them. The medical profession is broad, and catholic, and philosophic. Its aim is humanitarian, and it looks out with an eager eye into all the realms of nature and art, and wherever it finds any fact, or law, or principle, or method, or apparatus, or remedy, that can aid it in its noble work, it hails it with avidity, and presses it into its service with joy. It receives with gratitude any valuable suggestion, whether it comes from friend or foe. It goes upon the principle so humorously expressed by the celebrated Rowland Hill, when certain bigots rebuked him for joining with Unitarians in circulating the Bible: "I would receive the Bible," said he, "from his Satanic Majesty himself, if he would have the courtesy to hand it to me with a pair of tongs."

There is obviously, at the present time, a deplorable tendency among eminent scientists to a departure from the inductive process of reasoning, and a reckless indulgence in the wildest and most chimerical speculations. Darwin has built up a stupendous theory, which, according to his own admission, is not, and will not for millions of ages, be susceptible of proof. Huxley reluctantly confesses that there is not a single fact to establish the daring pretension of the vestiges of creation that matter can generate life, and yet he has what he calls a philosophic faith that if he could go back beyond all geologic periods to the regions of chaos and eternal night, his vision, sharpened, I suppose, by darkness visible, would behold the problem solved by the infant energies of ammonia and other gases. And thus, with one sweep of the imagination, would these men madly and impiously tear away the immovable foundations of historical and experimental evidence on which rests the sublime superstructure of the Christian faith. In like manner we see in the medical profession a disposition to indulge in loose deductions and vague theories, and thereby to array the discoveries of science against the indubitable facts of experience. The disuse of depletion in peritonitis, and the substitution of large doses of opium, which merely lessens the peristaltic motion of the intestines and relieves pain; the expectant and stimulating treatment adopted in pneumonia, on the ground that it is a self-limited disease, that the exudation in the second stage withdraws a pound or more of the solid constituents of the blood, and that counter-irritation interferes with the physical explorations of the chest; the abandonment of leeches, counter-irritants, and stimulating applications to the throat in diphtheria, because it is a constitutional affection, and the microscope has revealed the agency of germs in its production; and many other instances of a similar nature, all go to show a growing determination to place the art of medicine upon a fanciful instead of an experimental basis. The earnestness with which I protest against this innovation will, I trust, excite no surprise when it is known that, having through the whole course of my professional life refused to be guided by these false lights, and adhered to the fundamental principles in which I was educated, only modifying their application to meet the actual exigencies of disease, I have never lost a case of uncomplicated peritonitis, or diphtheria, and only one or two of pneumonia.

I once encountered an epidemic of scarlet fever, in which almost every patient was attacked at the outset with congestion of the brain, and death occurred in a few hours in every case in which depletion was not promptly employed. I was called, at that time, to see a child about two years old, who was in a state of unconsciousness, with flushed cheeks and intense heat in the head. Totally ignorant of the germ hypothesis, I opened the jugular vein and took from it two or three ounces of blood, and applied counter-irritants to the back of the head and neck, and recovery speedily followed without any unpleasant sequelæ. The avalanche of lore from the universities of Europe which is now coming upon us, threatens to carry away the last vestige of ancient and time-honored methods, and unless some powerful barrier shall be erected at once to check the tide of modern speculation, our hopes of immortality and our chances for holding on to this planet will be buried together in one common ruin.

> "O star eyed Science! hast thou wandered there
> To bring us back the tidings of despair?"

Dr. Elam, in the paper to which I have referred, has presented the subject under discussion in a strong light. He says:

"Science is knowledge, but such knowledge is not power in any practical sense. We know the motions of the planets, and can predict their phenomena with the utmost exactness, but we cannot influence them in any way. By science we know disease; science is diagnostic. It is by art that we treat it; art is therapeutic. All our art is derived from experience. It may be that in some few instances *a priori* considerations lead us to try certain modes of treatment; but, in general, they are empirical, and in all cases the final acceptance or rejection of the method is governed by experience. This could not be were medicine a science. Science knows, and is precise and positive. Art is variable, and selects. Science submits to no ignorance; but art is ignorant of much. Science is essentially contemplative; art is active. In the apt anti-thesis of Dr. John Brown, science puffeth up; art buildeth up. Practically, the result of this error of theory is this: With every advance of science we are too much disposed to think that an alteration in our art is necessary; otherwise we should be tacitly admitting the barrenness of the science. We forget the results of long experience, to run after the phantoms evoked by our improved knowledge. We make a discovery in chemistry or in microscopical science, and we are but ill satisfied if we cannot adapt it to our art. We improve in physiological knowledge; we learn the functions of a nervous tract with greater certainty; or we trace the relations of certain organs to extraneous influence more accurately; and, in accordance with this, we alter modes of treatment which, up to the present time, we have been accustomed to think and to find satisfactory. Our disappointment in the result does not always teach us wisdom for the future. I do not propose to enter deeply into the abstract question, but will merely state what I believe to be the fact, that pure science has in general done but little for art, while art has constantly and largely been contributing to the progress of science. In our profession this has eminently been the case; not the men of science, but those of careful and accurate observation, have generally been the men distinguished for healing gifts. Avoiding any allusions to men of the present day, let me illustrate my meaning by contrasting Harvey, the man of science, with Sydenham, the man of concrete observation; Sir Charles Bell, the discoverer, with Abercrombie, the physician.

"Medicine has the same relation to science that poetry or painting has; and inasmuch as the most complete knowledge of the laws of perspective and the theory of light and colors would fail to make a painter, or the most intimate acquaintance with the rules of versification would fail to make a poet, so the profoundest knowledge of physiology and of all the sciences tributary to medicine, would entirely fail to make a competent physician. Medicine is a faculty to be acquired, not a lesson to be learned—to be acquired by long and patient observation of complex phenomena, in their ever varying combinations—not to be reduced to the hard and inelastic formula of science. In itself, I reverence science; but in the interests of true progress and of humanity, I trust we shall, for the future, hear more of the art of healing, and less of the science of medicine."

I have thus frankly expressed my views with regard to the necessity for the infusion of new force and vigor into the practice of medicine; for the adoption of additional methods of treatment, and a most rigorous adherence to the lessons of experience. I believe that by this means alone we can arrest the downward tendency of the art, and restore the confidence of the people. I believe that by this means we can materially diminish the rate of mortality, and prevent, to a great extent, the occurrence of chronic disease. I believe, also, that by this means we can cure a large proportion of the chronic diseases which now exist. I admit, of course, that there are maladies which, in the present state of our knowledge, we cannot with certainty control. We do not understand the nature of the poisons of cancer or tubercle, nor have we antidotes for them. I have no doubt that in the progress of science we shall become enlightened upon both these points so unspeakably interesting and important to mankind. We cannot correct degenerations of tissue, or remove abnormal tissue when formed to any great extent, nor shall we ever be able to do so, unless some new faculty shall be developed within us whereby we shall be able to remove mountains or raise the dead. But for malaria, and the poisons of rheumatism, gout, rheumatic gout and syphilis, we have infallible antidotes, by means of which we can effectually eradicate them from the system. These poisons play a most prominent part in the production of chronic congestions, and it is exceedingly important to understand that these congestions are just as positive and obstinate as if they had been produced by other causes, and that they do not disappear in consequence of the removal of the poisons; but I maintain that they, and all other congestions of a chronic nature that exist independently of poisons, may, by a vigorous and persistent course of internal and external treatment, be radically and permanently cured, provided, as before intimated, that they have not gone to the extent of producing degeneration of tissue, or a considerable amount of abnormal tissue.

It is obvious that this definition includes in the category of curable affections a large proportion of chronic diseases, and if I am right, the propositions which I have laid down are fraught with beneficent consequences, the magnitude of which no language can exaggerate. They are, in opposition to the world wide scepticism, the proclamation of a gospel of faith and hope to all men, but especially to that great host of invalids who, like the woman in Scripture, have tried many physicians, and never grown better, but rather the worse, and who now, in weakness, or pain, or breathlessness, or all combined, are dragging out a wretched existence on bed or couch, in palace or hovel, or travelling up and down the earth in search of ease and rest, and finding none. Let it go forth as the blast of a trumpet that there is hope for them! Science is not powerless, but in her vast storehouse holds the treasures which will supply their wants. If her priests will only gird themselves for the work, and with wisdom and energy and perseverance employ the means which she puts at their disposal, then through all those ranks of sorrow and suffering will be heard a song of thanksgiving and praise.

I do not, of course, write in this manner without an adequate basis of facts. For the first fourteen years in which I was engaged in the practice of my profession I resided in Fredericton, the capital of the British Province of New Brunswick, a small town, now elevated to the rank of an ecclesiastical city, situated on the bank of a beautiful river, with a population embodying more varied and brilliant talent, intelligence and genuine kindheartedness, in proportion, than any other I have ever known. It is surrounded by an extensive country, in which my field of labor comprised a range of from thirty to fifty miles in different directions. During half the year the river and streams around are frozen over, and the ground is covered with snow, and sometimes the thermometer falls to thirty-six degrees below zero. At this season I travelled wrapped in furs, and sometimes in consequence of drifts I could only go at the rate of two miles an hour—a sorry pace for my patients who in pain or danger awaited my arrival. In the country there were no physicians to consult, and I was often confronted by the most difficult problems in medicine, and required to perform the most important operations, especially in obstetrics, without advice or assistance. It was necessary that I should be prepared for any emergency, and ready at a moment's call to execute any work, from the drawing of a tooth, or the removal of a button from a child's nose, to the amputation of a limb, the extraction of a stone from the bladder, or the management of a case of placenta praevia. When I came to this city, in 1850, I reported in the *New York Journal of Medicine and the Collateral Sciences* the first case, I believe, recorded in the United States of recovery from rupture of the uterus. Four years afterward I published in the *New York Medical Gazette* the report of a successful experiment in a remarkable case of ascites, by the introduction of air into the cavity of the peritoneum. During the last twenty years I have given special attention to the treatment of chronic diseases, and I am prepared to justify the claims which I have made in behalf of the great science to which I have devoted my life, by the presentation of successful cases in a series of papers, one on chronic rheumatism, one on asthma, and one on syphilis, to be followed by others in due time.

I cannot conclude this paper without a plea in behalf of that unfortunate class which, in addition to the sorrows and pains of hopeless disease, are forced to endure the pangs of poverty. Regarded by everybody as the victims of incurable evils, it was natural, perhaps, that little provision should be made for them, and that the dispensary system should be considered sufficient to furnish them with all the benefits which they could reasonably expect. But, I trust, when it shall be made to appear that there is no need of all this suffering and despair, and that they can be made whole and restored to their families and to society, that thousands of sympathizing hearts will rush to their relief and give them the aid which their condition imperatively demands. It has been the dream of my life to assist in founding a hospital for these helpless sufferers, and I am sure that there is not in the world an object of a charitable nature that is so urgently required. I need scarcely add that I am willing to give to it all the time and medical services which it would need from me, without further reward than the satisfaction I should feel in helping to carry forward such a noble enterprise. I have said that there is no such institution in the world. The establishment of the first would be a crowning glory to New York.

On the morning after the meeting of the association I received the subjoined note:

My Dear Dr. Hartt: I see by the morning papers that you read your essay last evening before the Medical Journal Association. I am sorry to say that a sharp attack of bronchitis kept me away. I regret it very much, for, besides the pleasure of hearing you again, I intended to say something in support of the views you advocate with such signal ability and eloquence. Believe me, my dear Dr. Hartt, with best wishes, most sincerely and truly yours,

J. Marion Sims.

267 *Madison Avenue, New York.*

CHAPTER II.

INDORSEMENT BY THE FACULTY.

After the presentation of the paper, I made a personal visitation of the medical Faculty of New York, and laid before them in detail my plan for the establishment of an institution in this city, on the broadest scientific and professional basis, for the treatment and cure of chronic diseases, and obtained for it the indorsement of a very large proportion of them, a catalogue of whose names I give in full.

The undersigned, members of the Medical Faculty of New York, recognize the necessity of the Hospital proposed by Dr. Hartt for the Cure of Chronic Diseases, both for the benefit of the poor who are suffering therefrom, and of the profession, as affording an opportunity to Medical Students to examine their nature and treatment. We, therefore, earnestly recommend the immediate establishment of such an Institution in this city.

J. Marion Sims, M. D., Founder of Woman's Hospital, and President of Am. Med. Association.

Alonzo Clark, M. D., Prof. Path. and Prac. Med. Col. Phy. and Sur., Pres. Fac., and Vis. Ph. Bel. Hosp.

Gurdon Buck, M.D., Vis. Sur. N. Y. Hosp., and Cons. Surg. to St. Luke's and Roosev. Hosp.

E. H. Davis, M. D., Ex. Prof. Mat. Med. N. Y. Med. Col.

B. W. M'Cready, M. D., Cons. Phy. Bel. and Charity Hosp.

Chas. A. Budd, M. D., Prof. Obstet. Med. Dep. N. Y. Univ.

John W. Draper, M. D., Prof. Chem., N. Y. Univ.

Martin Pain, M. D., Emer. Prof. Mat. Med. and Therap. M. D. N. Y. Un.

George A. Peters, M. D., Vis. Sur. N. Y. and St. Luke's Hosp.

Wm. H. Thompson, M. D., Prof. Mat. Med. and Therap., M. D. N. Y. Univ., and Vis. Phy. Roosev. Hosp.

John T. Darby, M. D., Prof. Surg. Med. Dep. N. Y. Univ.

Stephen Smith, M. D., Prof. Orthop., Sur. and Med. Jurisp. Med. Dep. N. Y. Univ.

THE COLUMBIAN INSTITUTE.

J. W. S. Arnold, M. D., Prof. Physiol., Med. Dep., N. Y. Univ.

Wm. A. Hammond, M. D., Prof. Dis. Mind and Nerv. System, Med. Dep., N. Y. Univ.

Oliver White, M. D., Cons. Phys. to Presb. Hosp.

Louis Elsberg, M. D., Prof. Laryng., Med. Dep., N. Y. Univ.

Montrose A. Pallen, M. D., Prof. Gynæcol., M. D. N. Y. Univ.

Wm. H. Draper, M. D., Vis. Phy. N. Y. and Roosev. Hosp., and Clin. Prof. Dis. Skin, Col. Phy. and Sur.

Fessenden N. Otis, M. D., Clin. Prof. V. D., Col. Ph. and Sur.

Jas. L. Little, M. D., Vis. Sur. St. Luke's and St. Vin. Hosp.

Alex. B. Mott, M. D., Prof. Clin. and Op. Sur. Bel. H. Col. and Vis. Sur. Bel. Hosp.

Jas. R. Leaming, M. D., Vis. Phy. to St. Luke's Hosp.

S. M. Cuyler, M. D., U. S. Army.

J. F. Hammond, M. D., U. S. Army.

F. O'Donohue, M. D., U. S. Army.

C. Sutherland, M. D., U. S. Army.

F. Zinsser, M. D., Memb. Med. Board, Germ. Hosp.

Lewis A. Sayer, M. D., Prof. Orthop. and Clin. Sur. Bel. Hosp., and Vis. Sur. Bel. Hosp.

R. Ogden Doremus, M. D., Prof. Chem. and Toxicol. B. H. Col.

G. M. Edebohls, M. D., House Ph. and Sur. to St. Francis' Hosp.

Max Herzog, M. D., Vis. Ph. Mount Sinai Hosp.

D. Froelich, M. D., Ph. and Sur. in Mount Sinai Hosp.

V. P. Gibney, M. D., Ass. Ph. and Sur., N. Y. S. for Rel. of Rup. and Crip.

J. J. Mason, M. D., Vis. Ph. Hosp. Epilep. and Paralyt.

Thomas Addis Emmet, M. D., Vis. Sur., Woman's Hosp., S. N. Y.

P. F. Mundé, M. D., Ass. Sur. and Ph., O. D. Dep., Woman's Hosp.

G. T. Harrison, M. D., Ass. Sur. and Ph., O. D. Dep. Woman's Hosp.

Bache McE. Emmet, M. D., Ass. S. and P., O. D. Dep., Woman's Hospital.

C. C. Lee, M. D., Ass. S. and P. O. D. Dep., Woman's Hosp.

Joseph E. Janvrin, M. D., Ass. S. and P., O. D. Dep., Woman's Hosp.

C. S. Ward, M. D., Ass. Ph. and Sur., O. D. Dep., Woman's Hosp.

H. L. Sims, M. D., Ass. P. and S., O. D. Dep. Woman's Hosp.

H. D. Nicoll, M. D., Ass. P. and S., O. D. Dep., Woman's Hosp.

J. N. Beekman, M. D., Pathologist, Woman's Hosp.

A. D. Rockwell, M. D., Electro Therap., Woman's Hosp.

Gustavus A. Sabine, M. D., Cons. Ph. Woman's Hosp.

Alpheus B. Crosby, M. D., Prof. G. D. and Sur. An., B. H. Col.

Henry D. Noyes, M. D., Prof. Opthal. and Otol., Bel. H. Col.

Jos. D. Bryant, M. D., Inst. P. and P. Med. Sur., and Ob. B. M. Col.

J. Lewis Smyth, M. D., Clin. Prof. Dis. of Child. Bel. H. Col.

W. Schirmer, M. D., Ex-Coroner.

S. B. Ward, M. D., Prof. Sur. Wom. Med. C., N. Y. Inf.

INDORSEMENT BY THE FACULTY.

J. W. S. Gouley, M. D., Vis. Sur. Bel. Hosp.

M. H. Henry, M. D., Sur. in Chief State Emig. Hosp.

Charles Phelps, M. D., Vis. Sur. St. Vincent's Hosp.

Joseph A. Kerrigan, M. D., Vis. Sur. St. Vincent's Hosp.

P. J. Clarke, M. D., Vis. Ph. St. Vincent's Hosp.

M. K. Hogan, M. D., Vis. Ph. St. Vincent's Hosp.

Thos. F. Healy, M. D., Vis. Ph. St. Vincent's Hosp.

C. H. Lellman, M. D., Vis. Ph. St. Francis' Hosp.

J. A. Tyndale, M. D., House Ph. and Sur. St. Francis' Hosp.

Henry L. Horton, M. D., Vis. Ph. Home for Incurables.

Wm. O. Moore, M. D., Res. Sur. Eye and Ear Infirmary.

R. Gebser, M. D., Ass. Sur. to N. Y. Ophth. and Aur. Inst.

G. W. Rachel, M. D. Clin. Ass. N. Y. Op. and Aur. Inst.

E. Blackwell, M. D., Emer. Prof. Hyg., W. M. C., N. Y. Inf.

G. H. Wyncoop, M. D., Prof. Phys., W. M. Col., N. Y. Inf.

E. H. Jaynes, M. D., Prof. Hyg. W., M. C., N. Y. Inf.

E. D. Hudson, M. D., Prof. P. and Prac. Med. in Wom. M. C., N. Y. Inf.

S. M. Roberts, M. D., Cl. Prof. Dis. Child., W. M. C., N. Y. Inf.

R. W. Taylor, M. D., Cl. Prof. Dis. Skin, W. M. C., N. Y. Inf.

Isaac Adler, M. D., Lect. on Path. Anat., W. M. C., N. Y. Inf.

J. W. Wright, M. D., Lect. on Minor Sur., W. M. C., N. Y. Inf.

L. D. Bulkley, M. D., Lect. on Med. Diagnosis, W. M. C., N. Y. Inf.

E. K. Henschel, M. D., Cur. Roosv. Hosp., and Lect. on Emerg., W. M. C., N. Y. Inf.

M. N. Baker, M. D., Cl. Ass., M. Clin., W. M. C., N. Y. Inf.

C. A. Loring, M. D., Cl. Ass. Skin Clin., W. M. Col., N. Y. Inf.

George G. Wheelock, M. D., Lect. on Phy. Diag., W. M. C., N. Y. Inf.

Robert F. Weir, M. D., Vis. Sur. Roosv. Hosp., and Lect. on Dis. Male Pelv. Organs., W. Med. Col., N. Y. Inf.

Woolsey Johnson, M. D., Vis. Phy. N. Y. Hospital.

H. F. Walker, M. D., Vis. Sur. Bel. Hosp.

Wm. M. Chamberlain, M. D., Vis. Phy. Charity Hosp.

F. R. S. Drake, M. D., Vis. Phy. Charity Hosp.

A. Kessler, M. D., Coroner.

H. Wakeman, M. D., Adj. Lect. Dis. Lungs and Pleura., B. H. Col.

T. H. Burchard, M. D., Adj. Lect. Dis. U. Tract.

J. J. Hull, M. D., Vis. Phy. Nursery and Child's Hosp.

James B. Reynolds, M. D., Vis. Phy. Nur. and Child's Hosp.

W. W. Jones, M. D., Con. Phy. N. and Ch. Hosp.

L. B. Joseph, M. D., Ass. Ph. N. and Ch. Hosp.

O. S. Payne, M. D., Sur. in charge St. Elizabeth's Hosp.

F. J. Bumstead, M. D., Cons. Sur. St. Elizabeth's Hosp.
W. M. Fleming, M. D., Cons. Phy. St. Elizabeth's Hosp.
W. L. Harding, M. D., Vis. Phy. Trinity Infirmary.
W. T. Bacon, M. D., Ass. Sur. Ophthalmic Department, Eye and Ear Inf.
P. A. Callan, M. D., Ass. Sur. Ophthal. Dep., Eye and Ear Inf.
W. S. Little, M. D., Ass. Sur. Ophthal. Dep., Eye and Ear Inf.
F. Simrock, M. D., Sur. Aural Dep., Eye and Ear Inf.
Albert H. Buck, M. D., Sur. Aural Dep., Eye and Ear Inf.
W. S. Ludlum, M. D., Sur. Aural Dep., Eye and Ear Inf.
C. McBurney, M. D., Vis. Sur. St. Luke's Hosp.
Andrew H. Smith, M. D., Vis. Phy. St. Luke's Hosp.
Clement Cleveland, M. D., Vis. Phy. Charity Hosp.
Edward Frankel, M. D., Vis. Phy. Charity Hosp.
Faneuil D. Weisse, M. D., Prof. Sur. Anat., M. D. N. Y. Univ.
Walter R. Gillette, M. D., Adj. Prof. Obst., M. D. N. Y. Univ.
Wm. Stratford, M. D., Adj. Prof. Chem., M. D. N. Y. Univ.
John T. Kennedy, M. D., Clin. Ass. Col. Phy. and Sur.
O. D. Pomeroy, M. D., Sur. Manh. Eye and Ear Hosp.
David Webster, M. D., Ass. Sur. Manh. Eye and Ear Hosp.
F. H. Rankin, M. D., Ass. Sur. Manh. Eye and Ear Hosp.

D. R. Ambrose, M. D., Ass. Sur. Manh. Eye and Ear Hosp.
Clinton Wagner, M. D., Vis. Phy. Metrop. Throat Hosp.
E. B. Bronson, M. D., Pathologist, Metrop. Throat Hosp.
J. Varnim Mott, M. D., Clin. Ass. Metrop. Throat Hosp.
D. H. Goodwillie, M. D., Clin. Ass. Metrop. Throat Hosp.
S. L. Griswold, M. D.
John Burke, M. D.
E. Noeggerath, M. D.
C. Bernacki, M. D.
L. Blumenthal, M. D.
Stephen de Wolfe, M. D.
H. F. Quackenbos, M. D.
John Bishop, M. D.
Thomas C. Finnell, M. D.
S. B. St. John, M. D.
Augustus G. Elliott, M. D.
J. L. Campbell, M. D.
W. C. Livingstone, M. D.
C. F. Taylor, M. D.
E. Heitzman, M. D.
S. McClellan, M. D.
John Hilton, M. D.
Joseph Worster, M. D.
E. F. Schwedler, M. D.
H. P. DeWees, M. D.
R. K. Colville, M. D.
A. Maclay, M. D.
T. Nichols, M. D.
G. M. Schweig, M. D.
W. G. Wylie, M. D.
F. M. Deems, M. D.
T. C. Chalmers, M. D.
J. P. Garrish, M. D.
F. L. R. Satterlee, M. D.
T. M. B. Cross, M. D.
W. W. Strew, M. D.

INDORSEMENT BY THE FACULTY. 41

E. W. Ranney, M. D.
J. O. Pond, M. D.
S. Fitch, M. D.
T. S. Bahan, M. D.
G. Z. Hunter, M. D.
A. H. Little, M. D.
B. F. Vosberg, M. D.
N. C. Levings, M. D.
J. W. Richards, M. D.
H. S. Gay, M. D.
T. A. Tellkampf, M. D.
H. L. Richardson, M. D
James O. Smith, M. D
H. T. Sears, M. D.
G. Bayles, M. D.
C. S. Wood, M. D.
A. S. Church, M. D.
E. Fowler, M. D.
G. B. Fowler, M. D.
S. R. Percy, M. D.
D. F. Fetter, M. D.
H. D. Ranney, M. D.
L. Weber, M. D.
Frederick Elliot, M. D
G. M. Beard, M. D.
H. M. Sell, M. D.
G. W. Brooks, M. D.
L. Ranney, M. D.
R. P. Lincoln, M. D.
S. R. Childs, M. D.
W. B. Neftel, M. D.
Jerome C. Smith, M. D.
A. Hodgman, M. D.
F. P. Kinnicut, M. D.
L. A. Rodenstein, M. D.
H. H. Gregory, M. D.
J. O. Farrington, M. D.
D. D. W. Harrington, M. D.
W. V. White, M. D.
J. Stachelberg, M. D.
E. Storer, M. D.

F. L. Harris, M. D.
T. M. Cheesman, M. D.
A. L. Ranney, M. D.
J. W. Warner, M. D.
W. P. Worster, M. D.
J. W. Brennan, M. D.
Wm. F. Fluhrer, M. D.
C. E. Nelson, M. D.
J. P. Garrish, Jr., M. D.
M. H. Williams, M. D.
E. G. Higginbotham, M. D
H. G. Forbes, M. D.
A. Tejeda, M. D.
F. Bedford, M. D.
W. Thurman, M. D.
G. H. Swezey, M. D.
W. C. Jordan, M. D.
W. M. Bullard, M. D.
S. D. Terry, M. D.
S. P. Vondersmith, M. D.
T. H. White, M. D.
E. Herrick, M. D.
F. A. Putnam, M. D.
S. Kelly, M. D.
A. S. Heath, M. D.
John C. Hannan, M. D.
H. E. Handerson, M. D.
C. E. Simmons, M. D.
N. Smith, M. D.
W. Schoonover, M. D.
J. B. McCaffrey, M. D.
B. A. Mylius, M. D.
S. Whitall, M. D.
A. Viele, M. D.
J. H. Fenner, M. D.
J. W. McWhinnie, M. D.
W. P. Ackerman, M. D.
D. C. Comstock, M. D.
J. R. Conway, M. D.
E. G. Rawson, M. D.
J. Dunn Stark, M. D.

S. Gluck, M. D.
K. Lampe, M. D.
J. Hoexter, M. D.
Charles F. Roberts, M. D.
James Moorhead, M. D.
James C. DeVerona, M. D.
D. F. Reynolds, M. D.
H. Obarius, M. D.
A. Kochler, M. D.
E. J. Darken, M. D.
J. W. Bowden, M. D.
S. K. Lyon, M. D.
D. B. Miller, M. D.
G. F. Carey, M. D.
E. Ilgen, M. D.
J. R. Van Kleck, M. D.
G. F. Friou, M. D.
Julius Frankel, M. D.
M. Michaelis, M. D.
Reuben Smith, M. D.
C. H. Avery, M. D.
G. L. Newcomb, M. D.
J. F. Ferguson, M. D.
M. C. Tully, M. D.
M. E. Tully, M. D.
H. G. Klotz, M. D.
L. DeBremon, M. D.
L. Conrad, M. D.
A. R. Strahan, M. D.
H. Von Seyfried, M. D.
B. Scharlau, M. D.
August F. Frech, M. D.
F. H. O'Neil, M. D.
S. H. Smith, M. D.
S. J. Henna, M. D.
T. M. Franklin, M. D.
J. H. Douglass, M. D.
C. Wright, M. D.
Albert D. Elmer, M. D.
W. M. Carpenter, M. D.
R. Taylor, M. D.

M. A. Wilson, M. D.
E. V. Agremonte, M. D.
F. G. Snelling, M. D.
H. R. Williams, M. D.
Jas. A. McLochlin, M. D.
C. G. Stanley, M. D.
A. A. Smith, M. D.
J. F. O'Connor, M. D.
Robt. Campbell, M. D.
A. A. Arango, M. D.
Frank L. Ives, M. D.
A. J. Minor, M. D.
F. S. Bates, M. D.
C. Imperatori, M. D.
L. B. Bangs, M. D.
C. A. Atwater, M. D.
T. E. Burtsell, M. D.
B. E. Hays, M. D.
T. J. Naughton, M. D.
Jas. J. Purcell, M. D.
John Purcell, M. D.
W. J. Welsh, M. D.
J. Nolan, M. D.
R. S. Prentiss, M. D.
Bernard Haran, M. D.
G. V. Hudson, M. D.
W. F. Thoms, M. D.
S. Hemingway, M. D.
E. J. Hogan, M. D.
A. Brandis, M. D.
A. J. Harrison, M. D.
I. D. Boehme, M. D.
T. J. Stout, M. D.
M. S. Buttles, M. D.
E. Lauer, M. D.
E. J. Messemer, M. D.
M. J. Messemer, M. D.
S. MacKiewicz, M. D.
A. Otterbourg, M. D.
Ellis S. Piercy, M. D.
J. Anderson, M. D.

INDORSEMENT BY THE FACULTY. 43

J. H. Anderson, M. D.
P. F. C. Deslandes, M. D.
J. C. Barron, M. D.
W. N. Campbell, M. D.
E. Boetzkis, M. D.
H. Hirschfield, M. D.
J. Neil, M. D.
John Shrady, M. D.
F. Muller, M. D.
L. Straus, M. D.
H. Lowenthal, M. D.
O. A. Rieffel, M. D.
C. E. Waechter, M. D.
G. C. Stiebling, M. D.
E. Wyler, M. D.
E. O. Cowles, M. D.
G. Treskatis, M. D.
C. A. T. Krog, M. D.
G. B. Hickock, M. D.
F. V. White, M. D.
E. D. Ramsdell, M. D.
J. R. Healey, M. D.
H. LeBaron Hartt, M. D.
A. E. Wettengel, M. D.
L. Schultze, M. D.
N. G. McMaster, M. D.
P. McDonald Allen, M. D.
J. C. Rising, M. D.
E. W. Lambert, M. D.
W. H. Maxwell, M. D.
C. W. Badeau, M. D.
J. R. Cypert, M. D.
E. W. Derby, M. D.
H. Williamson, M. D.
W. J. Purcell, M. D.
E. Hughes, M. D.
P. W. McDonnell, M. D.
R. C. Toseand, M. D.
Daniel Lewis, M. D.
G. L. Hyslop, M. D.
E. S. Finlay, M. D.

C. Milne, M. D.
C. Schneider, M. D.
Jas. W. Ranney, M. D.
C. T. Rodgers, M. D.
R. B. Burton, M. D.
R. G. L. Dieffenbach, M. D.
H. Peterhausen, M. D.
L. Putzel, M. D.
E. Rosenberg, M. D.
A. Hermann, M. D.
H. Assenheimer, M. D.
C. J. MacGuire, M. D.
J. W. Robie, M. D.
E. A. Maxwell, M. D.
I. F. Golding, M. D.
D. A. Leavitt, M. D.
A. Assenheimer, M. D.
M. Morris, M. D.
J. Mitchels, M. D.
L. Stern, M. D.
C. Roth, M. D.
H. Kost, M. D.
E. Petzold, M. D.
K. Bran, M. D.
H. L. Sheldon, M. D.
H. T. Strong, M. D.
G. F. Jackson, M. D.
W. Frothingham, M. D.
C. C. Cone, M. D.
M. Spicker, M. D.
A. S. Hunter, M. D.
J. T. Parker, M. D.
Daniel Cook, M. D.
George W. Holmes, M. D.
Ezra R. Pulling, M. D.
P. Burnett, M. D.
F. Walker, M. D.
J. C. Acheson, M. D.
J. B. Taylor, M. D.
J. Glaser, M. D.
Wm. Dwyer, M. D.

G. V. Skiff, M. D.
O. A. Lutkens, M. D.
I. G. Weber, M. D.
C. Kremer, M. D.
R. Fraenkel, M. D.
S. Callman, M. D.
M. M. Dunton, M. D.
H. F. Topping, M. D.
Francis Pinner, M. D.
C. Sherman, M. D.
W. Leech, M. D.
O. Sweeney, M. D.
E. S. Smith, M. D.
W. H. Virmylie, M. D.
A. V. B. Lockrow, M. D.
I. L. Wilson, M. D.
W. A. Conway, M. D.
Henry Raphael, M. D.
J. H. Leveridge, M. D.
J. N. Husted, M. D.
F. Nordeman, M. D.
Ira M. Lang, M. D.
N. Abbott, M. D.
D. E. McSweeney, M. D.
Wm. Newman, M. D.
M. C. O'Connor, M. D.
Nelson Place, Jr., M. D.
L. Feigenblatt, M. D.
O. J. Ward, M. D.
F. R. Newman, M. D.
Charles Brueninghausen, M. D.
I. H. Asch, M. D.
A. J. Rieffel, M. D.
L. Bopp, M. D.
A. Van Arsdale, M. D.
A. Krehbiel, M. D.
L. Weyland, M. D.
C. Meyer, M. D.
C. A. Nolden, M. D.
W. B. McGuire, M. D.
E. Waitzfelder, M. D.

A. Rose, M. D.
J. Scheider, M. D.
C. Atkinson, M. D.
A. C. Hutton, M. D.
C. E. Mohn, M. D.
M. Eisler, M. D.
A. Strong, M. D.
H. Hierthes, M. D.
H. Balser, Jr., M. D.
G. Thompson, M. D.
M. G. Raelfe, M. D.
R. C. Cone, M. D.
H. Sheppard, M. D.
J. Pfeiffer, M. D.
A. Murray, M. D.
D. Breckes, M. D.
E. T. Stutzer, M. D.
F. W. Lilienthal, M. D.
I. W. Greene, M. D.
Jos. Simrock, M. D.
W. J. Savage, M. D.
M. Hogan, M. D.
C. Miller, M. D.
H. E. Crampton, M. D.
C. F. W. Haase, M. D.
J. S. Thebaud, M. D.
P. J. Lynch, M. D.
A. Duberceau, M. D.
W. Balser, M. D.
A. Shutt, M. D.
R. A. Barry, M. D.
R. S. Chapin, M. D.
Henry Krollpfeiffer, M. D.
R. R. Gibbes, M. D.
A. Powell, M. D.
C. B. M'Questen, M. D.
G. H. Butler, M. D.
M. R. Vedder, M. D.
C. H. Greenough, M. D.
S. Hirsch, M. D.
J. Del Risco, M. D.

INDORSEMENT BY THE FACULTY. 45

George B. Packard, M. D.
H. Kahn, M. D.
G. W. Bull, M. D.
S. A. Mason, M. D.
E. Treusch, M. D.
J. G. Cardner, M. D.
J. O'Dwyer, M. D.
J. J. Reid, M. D.
W. A. Hawes, M. D.
F. Livermore, M. D.
E. Hall, M. D.
J. Cushman, M. D.
G. M. Arnold, M. D.
L. Schoney, M. D.
G. O. Morrison-Fiset, M. D.
W. H. Morse, M. D.
G. D. Bleything, M. D.
J. V. S. Wooley, M. D.
J. L. Terry, M. D.
C. M. Fairbrother, M. D.
A. Pramann, M. D.
H. A. C. Anderson, M. D.
L. Goldschmiedt, M. D.
J. Doran, M. D.
L. Lambert, M. D.
J. R. Macgregor, M. D.
J. L. Morrill, M. D.
F. A. Thomas, M. D.
C. Lyon, M. D.
P. V. Murray, M. D.
N. M. Freeman, M. D.
F. Bradnack, M. D.
W. Beach, M. D., ex-Coroner.
H. Kuenstler, M. D.
C. R. Ellison, M. D.
J. Dwyer, M. D.
D. C. Cocks, M. D.
H. T. Pierce, M. D.
W. O. Meagher, M. D.
C. J. Smith, M. D.
J. Wiener, M. D.

O. F. Jentz, M. D.
W. Schmidt, M. D.
D. Mandelbaum, M. D.
J. Hahn, M. D.
P. R. Schoenemann, M. D.
R. Muller, M. D.
E. S. Nichols, M. D.
Wm. Fernbach, M. D.
A. W. Maclay, M. D.
J. S. Monell, M. D.
C. P. Kreizer, M. D.
A. Kantrovitz, M. D.
D. McEwan, M. D.
C. A. Becker, M. D.
J. M. Andrews, M. D.
A. Lambert, M. D.
R. J O'Sullivan, M. D.
Stephen Wood, M. D.
L. D. Sproat, M. D.
R. Amabile, M. D.
C. Edell, M. D.
W. H. Farrington, M. D.
C. Y. Swan, M. D.
C. E. Denhard, M. D.
H. W. Good, M. D.
R. Linderwald, M. D.
F. L. Fisher, M. D.
G. W. Johnston, M. D.
Moritz Derleth, M. D.
N. S. Roberts, M. D.
T. H. Smith, M. D.
S. V. Pilgrim, M. D.
F. W. Spauger, M. D.
A. Steinach, M. D.
L. C. A. Knoth, M. D.
E. W. Burnett, M. D.
M. Bracker, M. D.
J. B. Vankleek, M. D.
G. W. Robinson, M. D.
John Robinson, M. D.
W. A. James, M. D.

J. W. Warth, M. D.
F. H. Weisman, M. D.
S. S. Bogert, M. D.
F. Mucke, M. D.
J. B. Campbell, M. D.
M. McLean, M. D.
Wm. O. Donnell, M. D.
P. Morrogh, M. D.
J. L. Colby, M. D.
G. Cosine, M. D.
A. N. Brockway, M. D
G. Steinert, M. D.
J. B. Read, M. D.
J. J. Ketchum, M. D.
Sam'l H. McIlroy, M. D.
J. J. Williams, M. D.
Henry Ruhl, M. D.
George L. Simpson, M. D.
J. E. Comfort, M. D.
J. L. Kennedy, M. D.
D. Grunhut, M. D.
J. H. Eden, M. D.
H. F. Hessler, M. D.
A. S. Dana, M. D.
J. Ross, M. D.
Geo. Riegel, M. D.
T. N. Hawkins, M. D.
H. S. Downs, M. D.
J. H. Dorn, M. D.
N. S. Westcott, M. D.
N. H. Drake, M D.
G. Lindsay, M. D.
T. H. Skinner, M. D.
W. F. Denning, M. D.
H. Walker, M. D.
Stephen G. Cook, M. D.
E. L Partridge, M D.
E. Denison, M. D.
G. M. Weeks, M. D.
E. F. Brush, M. D.
W. Stephens, M. D.

J. N. Merrill, M. D.
S. S. Bancker, M. D.
Hugh Mulreany, M. D.
P. E. Donlin, M. D.
J. F. Chauveau, M. D.
M. A. Finnell, M. D.
S. J. Clark, M. D.
M. E. Baldwin, M. D.
F. W. Tucker, M. D.
M. B. Early, M. D.
F. Fleet, M. D.
E. D. O'Neil, M. D.
G. R Morse, M. D.
L. Spanhake, M. D.
A. J. Chadsey, M. D.
T. B. Stirling, M. D.
B. C. M'Intyre, M. D.
Robert McNeilly, M. D.
B. Ruppe, M. D.
S. H. Dessau, M. D.
J. W. Clements, M. D.
S. N. Leo, M. D.
W. F. Cushman, M. D.
J. H. Wilson, M. D.
E. H. Van Winkle, M. D.
G. B. Parker, M. D.
G. Ceccarini, M. D.
H. Kudlich, M. D.
S. O. Hendrick, M. D.
F. D. Beane, M. D.
S. Ayres, M. D.
D. Matthews, M D.
O. G. Smith, M. D.
C. D. Sackett, M. D.
J. Hadden, M. D.
E. B. Warner, M. D.
J. T. Nagle, M. D.
G. Morraille, M. D.
B. M. Keeney, M. D.
K. Maclennan, M. D.
W. H. Ensign, M. D.

INDORSEMENT BY THE FACULTY.

S. W. Roof, M. D.
J. S. Carradine, M. D.
R. H. Sloan, M. D.
T. Steele, M. D.
D. Phillips, M. D.
E. Knight, M. D.
J. F. Saville, M. D.
T. H. Holgate, M. D.
G. Frauenstein, M. D.
D. A. Antonini, M. D.
J. Howe, M. D.
J. T. May, M. D.
W. May, M. D.
W. F. Osborn, M. D.
J. H. Comfort, M. D.
H. M. Cohen, M. D.
J. P. P. White, M. D.
S. B. W. McLeod, M. D.
A. F. Newman, M. D.
E. Herzberg, M. D.
R. J. McKay, M. D.
W. B. Edgar, Jr., M. D.
A. Rattray, M. D.
R. O. Mason, M. D.
J. A. Monell, M. D.
J. B. De Lendeta, M. D.
C. D. Varley, M. D.
Miles D. Nash, M. D.
W. H. Jackson, M. D.
H. P. Farnham, M. D.
W. M. Kemp, M. D.
Z. S. Webb, M. D.
E. Bradley, M. D.
E. T. T. Marsh, M. D.
P. B. Wyckoff, M. D.
L. A. Baralt, M. D.
R. A. Murray, M. D.
J. C. Morton, M. D.
E. M. Cory, M. D.
H. Gomez, M. D.
D. P. Austin, M. D.

C. M. Desvernine, M. D.
K. Reid, M. D.
J. S. Crane, M. D.
T. A. McBride, M. D.
J. E. Ramos, M. D.
T. M. Coan, M. D.
E. D. Simpson, M. D.
W. C. McFarland, M. D.
L. G. Doane, M. D.
U. G. Hitchcock, M. D.
N. B. Emerson, M. D.
R. S. Tracy, M. D.
K. Wylly, M. D.
C. Prince, M. D.
C. W. Bernacki, M. D.
M. Donnelly, M. D.
S. Kennedy, M. D.
A. Buchanan, M. D.
H. Griswold, M. D.
G. S. Winston, M. D.
S. S. Mulford, M. D.
G. W. Wells, M. D.
A. V. Brailly, M. D.
C. Brailly, M. D.
G. C. Arnold, M. D.
F. H. Hamilton, M. D.
G. Durant, M. D.
C. Dubois, M. D.
E. J. Villainy, M. D.
R. De Castro, M. D.
O. W. Armstrong, M. D.
H. McClain, M. D.
A. B. DeLuna, M. D.
C. W. Buchler, M. D.
D. A. Hedges, M. D.
C. M. Page, M. D.
C. McMillan, M. D.
E. Flies, M. D.
J. Cisneros, M. D.
S. Teller, M. D.
P. A. Morrow, M. D.

L. P. Walton, M. D.
R. H. Saunders, M. D.
R. J. McGay, M. D.
F. B. Lawson, M. D.
G. H. Fox, M. D.
H. B. Goulden, M. D.
D. C. Logue, M. D.
E. Vanderpool, M. D.
J. A. Williams, M. D.
J. Osborn, M. D.
J. Mulreany, M. D.
M. J. Moses, M. D.
A. Rowe, M. D.
Chas. Russell, M. D.
K. Tauszky, M. D.
Henry A. Miller, M. D.
S. Teats, M. D.
A. Lukins, M. D.
J. S. Lawrence, M. D.
C. Mackenzie, M. D.
S. A. Coon, M. D.
A. P. Dalrymple, M. D.
A. S. Jones, M. D.
L. F. Saas, M. D.
C. E. Lockwood, M. D.
W. J. Donor, M. D.
George Hart, M. D.
R. L. Miranda, M. D.
J. E. Whitehead, M. D.
H. Moeller, M. D.
E. F. Ward, M. D.
E. D. Morgan, M. D.
J. De W. Nelson, M. D.
L. Fisher, M. D.
J. S. Warren, M. D.
L. G. W. Limpert, M. D.
J. E. M. Lordley, M. D.
W. T. Nealis, M. D.
T. Roediger, M. D.
T. S. Furleigh, M. D.
W. H. Martin, M. D.

A. D. Hull, M. D.
W. M. McLaury, M. D
P. C. Cole, M. D.
A. A. Molony, M. D.
R. M. Fuller, M. D.
I. Hurdsfield, M. D.
A. W. Maynard, M. D.
G. P. Schirmer, M. D.
N. C. Husted, M. D.
C. Bliss, M. D.
Newton F. Curtis, M. D.
Valentine Brown, M. D.
S. A. Purdy, M. D.
K. R. Taylor, M. D.
C. Reincke, M. D.
W. Burns, M. D.
A. Eidenbenz, M. D.
G. W. Bigelow, M. D.
A. Ferry, M. D.
M. L. Mann, M. D.
J. M. Harvey, M. D.
F. Beach, M. D.
Chas. T. Whybrew, M. D.
G. Langmann, M. D.
W. H. Katzenbach, M. D.
M. Leo Woolf, M. D.
T. E. Clark, M. D.
W. S. Watson, M. D.
J. C. Thomas, M. D.
J. T. Taylor, M. D.
R. Newman, M. D.
J. C. Jay, M. D.
P. B. Porter, M. D.
B. Segnitz, M. D.
J. H. Kissam, M. D.
W. A. Ewing, M. D.
J. L. Turner, M. D.
E. C. Woodbury, M. D.
S. Waterman, M. D.
E. C. Harwood, M. D.
G. B. Bosley, M. D.

INDORSEMENT BY THE FACULTY.

J. H. Morgan, M. D.
A. Kesseler, M. D.
F. Marcinskowski, M. D.
W. E. H. Post, M. D.
J. W. Stronach, M. D.
W. Hasloch, M. D.
L. Demainville, M. D.
B. J. Byrne, M. D.
B. Thompson, M. D.
S. A. Raborg, M. D.
F. E. Hyde, M. D.
T. M. L. Chrystie, M. D.
J. Martin, M. D.
S. Caro, M. D.
J. H. Fruitnight, M. D.
A. A. Davis, M. D.

A. F. Liautard, M. D.
J. H. Dew, M. D.
J. H. McCreery, M. D.
S. D. Powell, M. D.
J. H. Steinau, M. D.
H. E. Owen, M. D.
C. Hitchcock, M. D.
W. B. Schuyler, M. D.
L. A. Stimson, M. D.
T. M. Calnek, M. D.
R. F. Clow, M. D.
L. Kohnle, M. D.
F. A. Utter, M. D.
J. E. Ferdinand, M. D.
D. W. Searle, M. D.

CHAPTER III.

INDORSEMENT BY THE CITIZENS.

A number of gentlemen of different professions who had become interested in the project, then addressed a letter to me, which I transcribe, requesting me to call a public meeting in its behalf.

HENRY A. HARTT, M. D.

Dear Sir: The time has fully come when your long proposed plan of a hospital for chronic cases should take some practical shape.

We venture, therefore, to suggest that you call at an early day, and some convenient place, a meeting of the many friends of the project, to consider what course may be best adapted to provide at once such a building as may serve for a commencement of your Institute for the Cure of Chronic Diseases.

Rev. T. M. Peters, D. D., St. Michael's Church, New York.
Daniel F. Tiemann, ex-Mayor of New York.
Rev. E. McGlynn, D. D., St. Stephen's Church, New York.
Rev. F. C. Ewer, D. D., St. Ignatius' Church, New York.
Rev. Stephen H. Tyng, Jr., D. D., Holy Trinity, New York.
Rev. Hugh Miller Thompson, D. D., Christ Church, New York.
Rev. Howard Crosby, D. D., Chancellor New York University.
Rev. W. Ormiston, D. D., Collegiate Church, New York.
Rev. Wm. M. Taylor, D. D., Broadway Tabernacle, New York.
Rev. George B. Cheever, D. D., Church of the Puritans, New York.
John A. Dix, ex-Governor of New York.
Hon. Wm. M. Evarts.
Ranald Macdonald.
J. Marion Sims, M. D.
E. H. Davis, M.D., ex-Prof. Mat. Med.
Rev. Morgan Dix, D. D., Rector of Trinity Church, New York.
Rev. Stephen H. Tyng, D. D., Rector of St. George's Church, New York.
Rev. Samuel Osgood, D. D.
Richard Kelly, President Fifth Nat. Bank, New York.
W. H. Wickham, Mayor of New York.
H. M. Peckham.
Rev. Richard S. Storrs, D. D., Church of the Pilgrims, Brooklyn.
Rev. J. Clement French, D. D., Pastor of Westminster Church, Brooklyn.

Wm. A. Darling, Pres. Murray Hill Bank, New York.
Daniel S. Martin, Professor Geology, Rutgers Female Coll., New York.
Peter Cooper.
Abraham S. Hewitt.
Jos. Worster, M. D.
Mark Blumenthal, M. D.
Chas. P. Daly, Chief Justice Supreme Court, New York.
Benj. N. Martin, Professor of Philosophy and Logic in New York University.
John K. Porter.
Daniel Curry, Editor *Christian Advocate.*
Grosvenor P. Lowrey.
Joseph H. Choate.
Everett P. Wheeler.
J. S. Newberry, M. D., Professor Geology, Columbia College, New York.
F. A. P. Barnard, President Columbia College, New York.
J. R. Brady, Justice Supreme Court, New York.
Rev. Wm. R. Williams, D. D., Amity Baptist Church, New York.

The meeting was held in Association Hall, and was very largely attended. Everett P. Wheeler, Esq., presided, and Geo. B. Hickock, Esq., M. D., was the secretary. I give the report of the proceedings with the addition of two or three letters that were omitted therefrom, which appeared in a newspaper at the time:

The president, on taking the chair, addressed the audience as follows:

Ladies and Gentlemen: I thank you for the honor of presiding at a meeting called for the purpose of taking the steps necessary to add another to those noble institutions which have done so much to relieve the sufferings of our common humanity. The City of New York is often reviled as the hiding place of fraud and crime. No doubt there is much need of reform in the great city we all love so well, but we can point with just satisfaction to the good works of charity and self-denying beneficence that are done every day in our midst, and beholding them, thank God and take courage. It may perhaps be doubted whether Christianity has yet accomplished much in making men more honest, and whether knavery is not as common here as it was in Rome two thousand years ago. But no one can deny that the religion of Christ has made men infinitely more humane. The poor, the old, the feeble, the blind, were thrust aside or trampled under foot by the strong and active in the heathen world. It was another teacher than any that Greece or Rome produced that taught men to build hospitals and homes for these unfortunates.

It is then in obedience to the precepts and example of the Saviour of mankind that our friend, Dr. Hartt, has united with many distinguished clergymen and physicians in calling us together to-night. I know it may be said he has a hobby. If the hobby be a good one, this is a topic for praise. No doubt many of the fine gentlemen in the court of Ferdinand and Isabella thought Columbus very tiresome; yet to them and to all he gave a new world. I admire Dr. Hartt's untiring energy and perseverance. He will lay before you the details of his plan, and it is for you and for the citizens of New York to crown it with well deserved success.

Two letters from gentlemen who had been expected to address the meeting, were then read by the Secretary:

From J. MARION SIMS, M. D., 267 Madison Avenue, New York.

To HENRY A. HARTT, M. D.

Dear Sir: I regret to say that circumstances beyond my control detain me from your meeting this evening. My sympathies are entirely with you in your noble effort, and I hold myself ready to help you in any way that I possibly can.

With best wishes for the success of your hospital movement, believe me, most truly yours.

From Rev. J. CLEMENT FRENCH, D. D., Pastor of Westminster Church, Brooklyn.

To RANALD MACDONALD, Esq.

Dear Sir: I have been hoping to be present at the meeting in Association Hall this evening, but an important adjourned meeting of our presbytery prevents. Yet I am anxious to send, thus, through you, my congratulations to Dr. Hartt for so auspicious an inauguration of the movement to establish a hospital for the cure of diseases generally called incurable.

I esteem the project worthy of the fairest field and the fullest favor.

My own interest in Dr. Hartt's proposed hospital arises directly from my knowledge of several cures effected by him which have almost baffled belief. Most notable of these is the case of Mr. Henry M. Peckham, formerly one of my most esteemed parishioners, now a member of Rev. Dr. R. S. Storrs' church. From the hour of my first acquaintance with Mr. Peckham, to the day in which Dr. Hartt undertook his case, he was one of the most continual and severe sufferers from asthma of the most aggravated type. This covers a period of at least fifteen years, which probably entitles it to be called a "chronic case." He has received for more than a year and a half past total relief, with no threat of recurrence of his torturing malady. The case of your son, also, is equally in point and conclusive. I am acquainted, moreover, with the cases of one or two gentlemen of the very highest standing, who have been cured by Dr. Hartt of chronic diseases — wretched sufferers with rheumatism and bronchitis. They are now vigorous, vivacious and voiceful.

Certainly such an institution as is proposed deserves success, and must engage the attention and interest of all who wait eagerly for deliverance from the body of these living deaths.

The secretary then proceeded to read the following documents:

Proposed institution for the radical and permanent cure of chronic diseases, such as rheumatism, gout, bronchitis, asthma, catarrh, fever and ague, dyspepsia, affections of the skin and nervous system, chronic congestions of the throat, spine, joints, and of the liver, kidneys, lungs and other internal organs, with every facility, in addition to other methods, for water in all its forms, medicated and unmedicated, the hot air bath, rubbing and passive motion, inhalation, electricity, electro-magnetism, galvanism and physical training.

This class of diseases is not generally admitted into our existing hospitals. I have devoted particular attention to them for many years, and believe in their curability in a large proportion of cases. I desire the coöperation of the clergymen, medical Faculty and benevolent capitalists of New York, in establishing an institution which will afford an opportunity for the more thorough study of these diseases, and in which all the agencies which modern science can command will be brought to bear for their entire and permanent cure.

HENRY A. HARTT, M. D.

From Rev. HORATIO SOUTHGATE, *D. D., Rector of Zion's Church, New York.*

There is evident need of such an institution as the foregoing plan proposes. It will be an invaluable addition to the numerous "Charities of New York." Everything seems to be provided for excepting "chronic diseases." Those our hospitals reject. This programme intends their cure. If it can be done, a new blessing is offered to our suffering humanity. If anyone can do it, he who has done it in numerous instances is the man. I, therefore, give my name as one who wishes to see the experiment tried under the most favorable auspices.

From Rev. EDW. MCGLYNN, *D. D., Pastor of St. Stephen's Church, New York.*

I cordially approve of Dr. Hartt's project of a hospital, and from the knowledge I have of his skill and humanity, on the testimony of those who have been cured, or wonderfully benefited in chronic cases, I am confident that the hospital would be a great public boon, especially to the poor.

From Rev. STEPHEN H. TYNG, JR., *D. D., Rector of Church of the Holy Trinity, New York.*

It gives me great pleasure to enroll myself among the friends of Dr. Hartt's new hospital. His extended experience and succes samong the class of chronic patients to whom its privileges will be offered, ensure the practical and effective administration of its interests when opened. I am confident that the project is worthy of all coöperation.

From Rev. GEORGE B. CHEEVER, D. D., *Pastor of the Church of the Puritans, New York.*

The proposed institution in this city cannot but be regarded as a most needed, important and beneficent undertaking. I most cordially add my commendation of the same; and having long known the ability and thoroughness of Dr. Hartt, in the treatment of such cases, I fully concur in the judgment so favorably expressed by others in behalf of such an establishment under his charge.

From Rev. HUGH MILLER THOMPSON, D. D., *Rector of Christ Church, Editor of Church Journal, New York.*

An institution like the one proposed is most desirable to crown the charities of our city, and, from all I know and believe, there is no man more competent to undertake it than Dr. Henry A. Hartt, a skilful and experienced physician, and an enthusiast in the study and treatment of a class of ailments which are generally left to the attention of advertising quacks, to the great injury and distress of the sufferers. Such an institution will also give to the medical student an opportunity now offered nowhere for the study of this class of diseases.

From Rev. THOMAS M. PETERS, D. D., *Rector of St. Michael's Church, New York.*

To HENRY A. HARTT, M. D.

Dear Sir: My interest in the object you have in view—the founding of a hospital for the treatment of chronic diseases—was long ago elicited by the enthusiasm animating you through many years of little encouragement from others. The hesitation to add to the number of our hospitals gives way before the *earnest recommendation* by so many of the eminent men of your profession, for the immediate establishment of such an institution. I shall gladly coöperate with and aid you, so far as it may be in my power.

From Rev. WILLIAM R. WILLIAMS, D. D., *Pastor of Amity Baptist Church, New York.*

The scheme of Dr. Hartt, for a great hospital in which chronic sickness may be effectually treated, seems to me full of promise, could it be sufficiently endowed; and with the attainments, character, and enthusiasm of its benevolent projector, and the blessing of God upon them, I should hope that the requisite funds may yet come from the wealth and generosity of our metropolis, which would find in such an institution one of its crowning adornments.

From Rev. CHARLES F. DEEMS, D. D., *Pastor of Church of the Strangers, New York.*

To HENRY A. HARTT, M. D.

Dear Sir: My intercourse with my brethren of the medical profession has been mostly in a social way, and, of course, I like them. When I shall need them professionally, who can tell? But if a man might make choice in such a matter, who would not choose to have many acute attacks rather than become a chronic sufferer? The very question shows what ground of appeal to our sympathies the chronic cases have. It will give me great pleasure to assist in your good work as I can; and may God prosper you!

From BENJAMIN N. MARTIN, *Professor of Philosophy and Logic in New York University.*

To HENRY A. HARTT, M. D.

Dear Sir: I desire to express to you hereby more formally than I could do in our conversation of a few days since my earnest sympathy in your proposal for a hospital for chronic diseases. The victims of such diseases are unquestionably numerous, and they are often unable to obtain proper treatment themselves, while they are of necessity excluded from our ordinary hospitals. Humanity, therefore, seems absolutely to require that some provision should be made for their necessities. The enlarged opportunities, moreover, which such an institution must afford for the study of such diseases in all their varied forms, constitute an additional and important recommendation of it.

I rejoice, therefore, that you have brought before the profession, and propose to bring before the public, the urgent need which exists for the establishment of such a hospital, and the great advantages which may be derived from it.

I feel personally grateful to you for your laborious efforts in this behalf, and shall cordially coöperate with you in every practicable endeavor to secure the founding of so benevolent and useful an institution.

From Rev. F. C. EWER, D. D., Rector of St. Ignatius' Church, New York.

I have known Dr. Henry A. Hartt for a number of years, and have had an opportunity of witnessing the successful results of his skill in several cases of chronic rheumatism, asthma, and nervous affections. His project of establishing a hospital (which now seems likely to be crowned with success) is, it seems to me, wise and beneficent, and eminently deserving of liberal practical encouragement.

From long experience I can testify, and I take pleasure in doing so, that there is no class of citizens who give more willingly and liberally of their time and valuable help to the poor than the medical profession.

The institution which Dr. Hartt proposes would not only confer an incalculable benefit upon those who are in the double misfortune of chronic disease and poverty, but it would furthermore cheer the hearts of thousands in the medium and upper walks of life, who having tried innumerable remedies, and gone from place to place in vain efforts for relief, have at last settled, hopelessly and exhausted in patience and purse, into what seems to be some incurable disease.

From Rev. W. ORMISTON, D. D., *Pastor of Collegiate Church, New York.*

To HENRY A. HARTT, M. D.

Dear Sir: In view of the unanimity with which so great a number of the medical gentlemen of this city speak of the necessity of such an institution as you propose, having also heard your own statements with reference to it, and believing that such a hospital would be a priceless boon to many a hopeless sufferer, I most heartily wish you all success in procuring the means and support requisite for its establishment. And I feel assured, if the wisdom of experience and the fervor of enthusiasm can command success, you need not fear failure.

From Rev. HOWARD CROSBY, D. D., *Chancellor of the New York University.*

It gives me great pleasure to add my testimony to the need of a hospital for the relief and cure of chronic diseases and to the personal worth of Dr. H. A. Hartt, whom I have known for many years. I trust his earnest efforts in behalf of so important a charity will be speedily crowned with success.

From Rev. R. S. STORRS, D. D., *Pastor of Church of the Pilgrims, Brooklyn.*

Dr. Hartt's plan for his proposed hospital appears to me most wise, practical, and beneficent. I am personally acquainted with some of those to whom he has rendered great and permanent service; and I not only wish him success, but will gladly do anything in my power to secure and further his success in the grand Christian work which he has now taken in hand. It seems to me one of the best that has ever been brought to my notice.

From Rev. E. S. WIDDEMER, *Pastor of the Church of the Reconciliation, New York.*

DEAR DR. HARTT:

It is really with great pleasure that I write to express my

thanks for what your medical skill has done in curing me of that horrible disease, dyspepsia. You will, I doubt not, remember how utterly faithless I was in your ever helping me when I first came to you, for it seemed to me I had tried almost everything in the *materia medica*. I am now firmly and fully convinced through my own experience, that your project for establishing a hospital for the treatment of chronic diseases is one of the greatest necessities of the age. It seems to me it would pay even if it were only to cure dyspeptic clergymen.

From GEORGE JONES, ESQ., *Proprietor of the New York Times.*

To Rev. J. CLEMENT FRENCH, D. D.

Dear Sir: I went to Dr. Hartt for rheumatic gout, which he treated with great success. Of this I can speak very emphatically. Some friends also tell me he was equally successful with them in asthma, and bronchial affections, and I should recommend him in these cases without hesitation. I should go to him were my rheumatic difficulty to return, with much confidence in his skill and ability to relieve me. I can further say the doctor seems devoted to his profession, and desirous to relieve those who cannot pay as faithfully as those who can.

From RANALD MACDONALD, ESQ., *33 Second Place, Brooklyn, New York.*

My son had been painfully afflicted with asthma for fifteen years, and instead of outgrowing it he continued getting gradually worse, being at last confined to the house about half of his time. He was at the worst stage of his disease when placed under Dr. Hartt's care in November, 1874, when, after the first few days his asthma disappeared, and strength came gradually. He has continued free from asthma, and is now regarded as permanently cured. The laudable desire to found in New York a hospital for the treatment and cure of chronic diseases has my heartfelt sympathy. I believe it will be the crowning glory of New York's great works of benevolence, and a lighthouse of charity, cheering the hopeless sufferers of our own vicinage while pointing the way to similar enterprises throughout the Christian world.

From URIAH WELCH, ESQ., *Proprietor of the St. Nicholas Hotel, New York.*

I have the greatest confidence in Dr. Hartt as a physician. I received the greatest possible benefit from his treatment, and after having suffered severely from both catarrh and asthma for a very long time, am now greatly or entirely free from both. I have entire faith in the efficacy of his treatment. * * * My sister called upon Miss Margaret Bloxham, at her residence, in Charlestown, Mass. She stated that she had had the asthma in its worst form for eight years, accompanied all the time by incessant cough, and that she was unable to sleep in a recumbent position day or night. She was so perfectly cured by Dr. Hartt that she had had no return of the disease for eight years, although residing the greater part of this time in the place where it was contracted. This note is only for use in the efforts to establish a hospital for the cure of chronic diseases, an institution much needed, and which I hope to see established on a solid basis at no distant day.

From STEPHEN DE WOLFE, M.D., *138 West Thirty-seventh Street, New York.*

To HENRY A. HARTT, M. D.

Dear Sir: Your paper on the "Prevention and Curability of Chronic Diseases" is one admirably calculated to awaken the profession to the necessity of again resorting to those measures so successfully used by our forefathers. Knowing, as I have for some years, your enthusiastic devotion to the treatment of chronic diseases, I am surprised that a hospital has not been opened before this for poor unfortunates suffering therefrom, with you at the head of it. I hope ere long the dream of your life will be realized in the successful operation of such an institution. It only needs the wealth and influence of large hearted New York once enlisted in its favor to make it all your fondest aspirations could desire.

From FRANK H. HAMILTON, M. D., *43 West Thirty-second Street, New York.*

To H. A. HARTT, M. D.

Dear Sir: I take pleasure in saying to you that your plan for the erection of a hospital for the treatment of chronic maladies meets my cordial approval.

From Prof. E. H. DAVIS, M. D., *175 East Eighty-second Street, New York.*

To H. A. HARTT, M. D.

Dear Sir: I have seen your proposed plan of a hospital for the cure of chronic diseases, and am satisfied of the importance of such an institution for the accommodation of a class of sufferers not generally admitted into the existing hospitals. Your thorough medical education, long experience, and enthusiastic devotion in the treatment of chronic diseases, especially fit you for the accomplishment of this great object. I have seen and examined several patients who have been treated by you for chronic rheumatism, asthma, and other affections, have been greatly pleased and surprised by the results I have witnessed, and am satisfied that your pretensions with regard to the cure of chronic diseases are well founded.

From the late Prof. CHARLES A. BUDD, M. D., *New York.*

Understanding that it is in contemplation to establish an institution in this city, for the special care and treatment of chronic diseases (usually regarded as incurable), I take pleasure in stating my conviction of the necessity of such an asylum, as many of our existing hospitals utterly refuse admission to this class of patients.

From Prof. JOHN W. DRAPER, *New York University.*

DR. HARTT.

Dear Sir: You can add my name to your hospital list.

The chairman then called upon Dr. Hartt, who delivered the following address:

Mr. Chairman, Ladies and Gentlemen: I have purposed for several years, with the help of God, and of the medical faculty and benevolent capitalists of New York, to establish a hospital in this city, exclusively for the treatment and cure of chronic diseases. I had long witnessed the deplorable neglect and mismanagement of these difficult and intractable maladies, both by private practitioners and public institutions. I had seen that the general hospitals, for the most part, rejected them by rule, while those connected with the Department of Charities and Correction, though obliged by law to provide for them, were totally destitute of some of the most important agencies and instruments which are absolutely necessary for their proper treatment, and, as a matter of fact, received them, in a large proportion of cases, with the view of affording temporary relief, rather than for the purpose of effecting a radical and permanent cure.

I began this undertaking with an effort to enlist the sympathy and coöperation of eminent clergymen in this city. The result, thus far, has been laid before you.

My second step was the preparation of a paper on the "Prevention and Curability of Chronic Diseases," which was read before the Medical Library and Journal Association. It was designed to embody a summary of my views with regard to the alarming prevalence of these diseases; the various causes which had led thereto; and the methods which should be adopted to effect their prevention and cure. It was received with marked dissatisfaction by the younger members of the association, but tokens of sympathy and approval were sent to me by physicians of age, and experience, and high. standing, in different parts of the country, and touching appeals for aid, and prayers for the hospital, came from helpless sufferers, who had long languished in despair, yet over whose dreary path I had fortunately been able to cast a ray of hope.

My third step was a personal appeal to the medical Faculty of New York. I thought that they would naturally be regarded as the rightful and authoritative judges in this matter, and that their decision would be final and absolute. I know it was considered an adventurous course to pursue, immediately after the publication of a stringent criticism upon modern practice. But I understood too well the common sense and acuteness of my brethren to suppose that they could fail to perceive, that a man who had been silently engaged for twenty years in the discovery and accumulation of facts, would not be likely to come out at the end of that period for mere selfish purposes; and I was persuaded that they were too fair minded and just to condemn him for the frank and honest expression of his opinions, whether right or wrong. Sir, I wish I could convey to you, in adequate language, my appreciation of the kind and courteous manner in which I have been received, and of the promptitude and cordiality with which my proposition has been accepted, by the great body of the profession in this city. Whatever shall be the fate of my enterprise, I shall ever look back with pride and pleasure to the incidents of this visitation. I have met, of course, in some few instances, with coldness and opposition. To those who differ from me substantially on the merits of the question, I freely concede the right to their opinion; while to those who dissent on other grounds, I bear only good will; and to each and all, from my heart, I give the right hand of fellowship.

It has been the custom, from time immemorial, to imagine that the medical profession is limited to a few remedies and appliances. When the heroic system prevailed, its range of therapeutics was supposed to be restricted, for the most part, to a certain routine of antiphlogistic measures;

and since, through the luxurious habits of society and homœopathy combined, the fashionable style of treatment has assumed the expectant form, anæsthetics, restoratives, opiates and sedative poisons have been considered almost the sum total that its legitimate resources can supply.

Meanwhile quackery, with its keen eye, has seen its advantage, and seizing here one important agency, and there another, has pretended with each single handed and alone, to cure every class and variety of disease. Who can tell the multitudes who have suffered on in life long agony and despair, and the still greater multitudes who have gone down to an untimely grave in consequence of this deplorable delusion? I will not presume to say how far the Faculty themselves are responsible for these calamities. But the time has come when they should assume their true attitude; when they should apply to their science the motto of the immortal Shakespeare: "Books in the running brooks, sermons in stones, and good in everything;" and when, as the undisputed successors of the apostles of medicine, they should peremptorily claim that every remedy, appliance, and instrumentality, from whatever department of nature or art they come; whether discovered by the learned or the unlearned; whether presented by the hand of savage or sage; whether wrought out in crucibles and retorts or manufactured in workshops; whether derived from the wilderness or the meadow, from the mountain or the rock, from the ocean or river or fountain, or from the mysterious powers of the air; all belong by an indefeasible right to them, and that they are bound to employ them separately or in combination, under the direction of common sense and medical knowledge, for the benefit of suffering humanity. By this means they would blot out at once and forever, not as scientific methods, but as systems of charlatanism, both hydropathy and the Swedish movement cure; and if, in the spirit of the age in which we live, they would go still further, and *casting down the middle walls of partition, affirm the equal rights of all thoroughly educated medical men, and trust to the power of free thought and free discussion for the correction of error and the advancement of truth,* I feel assured it would not be long before homœopathy and eclecticism, as distinct schools, would disappear, and there would be a general union and brotherhood over which the whole earth would have reason to rejoice.

In the medical profession, as in the church, there is a variety of gifts. Some prefer one department and some another; some affections of the eye, others of the ear, some surgery, others obstetrics, some lunacy, others the diseases of children, and one gentleman said to me: " I do not care, sir, for your institution, or for humanity. I treat one class of diseases only. My friends have furnished me with a dispensary, and so long as they give me plenty of money to carry it on I am satisfied. There are just two things in this world I love; one is skin diseases, the other is fishing. To-morrow I'm going to fish." I told this anecdote to a facetious friend, who said: " It must be admitted that he's a scaly fellow, anyhow." The treatment of chronic diseases requires a peculiar mental and moral constitution, and it would be just as impossible to find in every physician a man adapted to this particular field as it would be to find in every clergyman a brilliant orator, in every lawyer an able jurist, in every scientist a profound logician, or in every student of literature a magnificent poet. The grand qualifications for this sphere of labor are grit, patience, energy, and the irresistible magnetism of an unconquerable faith.

It is a matter for grave consideration, whether the influence of political and medical clubs forms a safe element in appointments to office, even in hospitals for acute diseases; but in the institution I propose it would obviously prove utterly and irremediably disastrous. The selection must be made sacredly with reference to the absolute fitness of every man for his post; and all should be chosen for life or during good behavior; and I consider it a point of great importance that there should be on the staff a scientist endowed with genius and thoroughly equipped by previous training and discipline, who should confine himself exclusively to the work of investigation, and whose aim should be by chemical analysis and microscopic examination to aid his colleagues in their intricate cases, and to make discoveries which would materially increase our knowledge both with regard to diseases curable and incurable. It would be difficult to conceive a grander theatre for research than would be afforded by an institution of this description; and chiefly with a view to this object, I would decidedly advocate the admission of many cases of cancerous and tubercular affections in their incipient stages, although properly classed among incurable diseases, because they constitute such admirable subjects for further study, and infold such splendid possibilities for the advancement of medical science. If, perchance, the effect of our labors should be, directly or indirectly, immediately or remotely, to solve the problem of the true nature and treatment of these malignant and destructive maladies, it alone would repay a millionfold our sacrifices and our toils.

The peculiar methods of this institution I propose to throw open to the whole Faculty of New York, for the benefit of their office patients. In this way every physician in the city would have at his command all the special appliances which he requires for the cure of chronic diseases, to be used by experts in accordance with his instructions, and under the rules of the most delicate professional etiquette.

Sir, a question has been raised with reference to the rights of medical men in our system of hospital management, the discussion of which is not only pertinent to this occasion, but is irresistibly forced upon me, because in the position which I occupy—a position which I have voluntarily assumed—I am bound in honor to make myself distinctly understood upon this point, and to be as frank and explicit in the expression of my opinion thereon in my appeal to the capitalists, as I was in the declaration of my views upon medical subjects in my appeal to the Faculty. I have seen in the newspapers an account of a remarkable transaction on the part of a Sister of the Poor of St. Francis, in St. Peter's Hospital, Brooklyn, who ordered its medical officers to discontinue a course of lectures, forbade the attendance of their brethren to witness their operations, and summarily ejected the house physician.

A still more flagrant instance of arrogance and wrong has occurred. The founder of a great institution—a man whose name will be held in imperishable honor, and cherished in the loving and grateful hearts both of men and women throughout the civilized world to the remotest ages—like Lear, has been virtually expelled by his daughters from the house which his own hands had built. Is there any reason to believe that there would be a hospital for woman in the world to-day, were it not for the inventive genius and generous heart of Marion Sims?

It was said that he made an unguarded and untimely speech. I will not ask an apology from him on this account. On the contrary, I admire him the more that when he heard of an insult offered to an honorable colleague, arising out of a rule which in itself involved an interference with the rights of his profession, in the heat and excitement of a just indignation he could not pause to weigh with accuracy the force of his language, or to adjust it with nicety to the measure of his own personal interests. I am convinced that, if the nature and extent of this outrage were understood by the Faculty of New York, they would rise in their majesty and demand with a voice of thunder that this beloved and celebrated brother should be forthwith restored to his place on the staff, of which, without disparagement to the eminent abilities and services of his former associates, he must ever be regarded as the rightful and natural head.

I confess that I am astounded at these revelations. What has the medical profession done that its most distinguished members should thus be subjected to the whims and caprices of lady superintendents, and ignominiously dismissed by governing boards? Preëminent, as a class, for their intelligence and culture, habitually devoted to the cause of science and the interests of humanity, I confidently assert their equality, by virtue of their office and character, with the highest and noblest citizens of this or any other country. By what authority or on what principle shall this discourtesy to them be defended? You admire and applaud the heroes who protect your honor and your homes on the battle field. Should you not love and reward yet more the men, who, without the pomp and circumstance of war, for you and for those who are dear to you, expose themselves continually to the still greater danger of the "pestilence that walketh in darkness?" The services they render, the sacrifices they make, the anxieties they bear, can never be adequately repaid. In all your sorrows they sympathize, in the hour of peril they cheer you, and when death comes at last they watch over you, and smooth your passage to the tomb. In no circumstance and under no consideration, not even to secure the highest object of ambition, would I falter in my duty to them, or fail to uphold with all my energies their dignities and their rights. I hold immovably to the opinion that, in every hospital, the physicians and surgeons connected therewith should be *ex-officio* members of the governing board, with full powers to act on all questions, financial or medical. As far as the interests or necessities of patients are concerned, they would go to the full extent of a just liberality, but in all matters merely of taste and ornamentation they would be frugal and conservative, and I venture to affirm with the utmost certainty that they would never consent to the purchase of a palace to be used as a club-house for themselves and their associates.

A voice of sorrow, a wail of anguish and despair from every quarter comes to us; from town and country, from rude hamlet and ruder tenement it comes, beseeching for help. O! if I could bring before you in one vast panorama a view of these pitiable sufferers; if I could show them to you tossing to and fro in agony, or gasping convulsively for breath, or lying forlorn and disconsolate under the pressure of a hopeless paralysis, cursing the day they were born, or praying devoutly to heaven for patience and resignation, your hearts would overflow with sympathy, and you would feel that your treasures were worthless, except in so far as they could administer to the relief or removal of this intolerable woe! I know that there is a class of men, even in this age of light and civilization, who regard all such considerations as the indications and ebullitions of a weak sentimentalism; who will point you to the old Spartan law which decreed that deformed children should be put to death, and who will exultingly refer you to the Darwinian theory of the survival of the fittest. I am glad when infidel scientists and their disciples stand thus fairly upon their own ground and push their speculations to their legitimate conclusions. It is well the world should know that when they take from us the Bible and declare that God is unknown and unknowable, they naturally and inevitably remit us to all the cruelties and barbarities of ancient Paganism.

Christ pronouncing beatitudes on the mount, healing the lepers, and curing all manner of diseases among the people, and on the cross, with divine compassion, praying for his murderers; and Paul, on Mars' Hill, proclaiming the universal brotherhood of man, afford alone to the popular mind and heart a sufficient answer to these wild and savage hallucinations; and while these two sublime figures shall be recognized in history, the rights of human nature will be protected and its sorrows assuaged.

In the name, then, of this great army of sufferers I come to you for aid. I ask you to join with me in a grand effort to deliver them from their terrible afflictions. What higher honor or privilege could we desire in life than to be allowed to consecrate our talents, our energies, and our wealth to an object of such transcendent importance? The pursuits of knowledge, and fame, and riches, under the guidance of an honorable ambition, are fitly attended with pleasure; but that pleasure is as a drop to the ocean, or as a spark to the full blaze of the meridian sun, when compared with the joy that springs from the exercise of Christian benevolence. I have always thought that one of the strongest arguments in favor of the inspiration of the Scriptures is that they give to God the title of Love, and represent it as the eternal fountain of happiness to him, and to all created intelligences. By the sacred authority, benign influences, and ineffable rewards of this great central force of the moral universe, I implore you to hail with delight the opportunity which I offer you, and to begin with me this day a work which will prove a perennial source of enjoyment to ourselves, and which will be attended with measureless benefits to the world for many generations.

E. H. Davis, M. D., spoke as follows:

Mr. Chairman: It might seem presumptuous in me to make any remarks on the importance of the hospital after listening to the eloquent and learned gentlemen who have preceded me. And I assure you I would not attempt it were it not that I am in possession of a few facts essential to the success of the project. I wish to say a word to my professional brethren who, like myself, have been more or less sceptical on the subject of the general curability of chronic diseases, such as asthma, rheumatism, dyspepsia, etc. I must confess that when Dr. Hartt first proposed his plan of a hospital for this purpose, and stated that a large percentage of such cases could be radically and permanently cured, I at least thought him an enthusiast, and my caution led me to withhold my approval until I had thoroughly investigated his cases, and fully satisfied myself of the facts. I now consider it my duty, both to him and to the profession, to state the result of my observation. I have examined, during the past two years, some ten or twelve persons treated by him for asthma, chronic rheumatism, and dyspepsia. Many of the cases represented the most serious types of the respective diseases, and had existed from two to thirty-five years. I do freely admit that I have been pleased and surprised by the results I have witnessed, particularly with regard to their uniformity and permanence, and I am satisfied that his views with reference to the curability of chronic diseases are well founded. The doctor makes no concealment with respect to his treatment, nor does he use secret remedies. His methods are altogether legitimate and purely scientific, and he intends to lay them before the profession, without reserve, as soon as practicable. One of his principal reasons for wishing the immediate establishment of the hospital is that it will afford him great facilities for demonstrating the correctness of his views, and the effectiveness of his plans of treatment. He has spent a large portion of his professional life in the study and treatment of this class of diseases, and it would seem strange, indeed, if, with his powers of observation and analysis, his large experience, implicit faith, and great enthusiasm had not resulted in the adoption of new combinations and applications of methods and remedies to achieve success. I have the honor of being intimately acquainted with a large number of medical men, and I say with confidence, I know no man whose heart beats more loyally to his profession, or who would shrink with greater repugnance from the thought of violating what he believed to be its established code of ethics. He has made great sacrifices in order to obtain important facts for the benefit of science and humanity, and I think the profession at large, who have already treated him with such marked kindness and consideration, will allow him great latitude in the selection of his own time and method to make known the result. It may be said, without any intention to flatter, that all who know Dr. Hartt must admit that he possesses, in an eminent degree, those qualities which fit him for carrying on this great work of charity. I close by hoping he may receive from capitalists that substantial aid which will enable him to establish the institution in accordance with his ideal, and so attain the object of the long cherished wish of his life.

Speech of Chancellor Crosby:

Mr. Chairman: I have listened with great pleasure to the forcible and eloquent address of Dr. Hartt, and have been interested in every part of it and fired by some. A great deal is said about New York being a very wicked city. I think it is the best abused city in the world. I say and challenge contradiction, having visited very many large cities, that New York is a clean city, and will bear comparison with any of its sister cities on this or any other continent. And against all that is said of its depravity and corruption, I assert that New York is a moral city. The trouble is that all its vices are given to the world, while but little publicity is given to its virtues. The other day a most horrible murder was committed not far from here, and two columns of a daily paper were devoted to its frightful details. The same day a little child crossing the ferry, near the same spot, fell into the water, and was saved from drowning by a brave and noble man, who risked his life, David Jordan—let his name be shouted—David Jordan! And how much space do you suppose was given to this incident in the same paper? Five lines! Two columns to the brutal murder, and five lines to the heroic act! With regard to the medical aspect of this question, I know nothing; but when I see so many eminent physicians giving it their support, I do not hesitate. I am now engaged in revising the translation of the Bible. And when we, in that work, find Sinaitic, Alexandrian, and Vatican manuscripts agree, we accept the text as unquestionable. So when, in a medical matter, Dr. Alonzo Clark, Gurdon Buck and Charles Budd lead, I am not afraid to follow. One thing I can say, that, having known Dr. Hartt for many years, I believe he would make a good leader in any cause. A feature which, I confess, brings this matter within my perfect sympathy is that it is a charity, in which all sects and denominations can meet on common ground.

The Rev. Dr. McGlynn having, by mistake, been introduced as a member of the medical profession, spoke in substance as follows:

This is not the first time that this mistake has been made. Once when I was called to administer spiritual comfort to an old woman who was sick, she told me all about the symptoms of her disease, and, on my assuring her that I knew nothing at all about medicine, she replied: "I know that you're a doctor as well as a priest, and if you only would you could tell me all about it." Though I have not the honor to belong to the medical Faculty, yet I do not by any means feel out of place on this platform, as a minister of him who went about doing good, and healing all manner of sickness among the people. It is in its aspect as a work of benevolence that I want to speak a word in favor of the institution proposed by Dr. Hartt. There are in this city and all over the country multitudes of sufferers, like the man who had an infirmity thirty and eight years, and who sat at the Pool of Bethesda waiting for an angel to move the waters; and when a good angel in the person of Dr. Hartt comes to their relief, we ought to welcome him with our sympathy and support. Let us never forget that it is by the performance of such works of Christian charity that our characters shall be judged, when our Saviour shall say, "Inasmuch as ye did it unto one of the least of these my brethren, ye have done it unto me." From the testimony of many who have been cured by the doctor, and from personal experience of treatment at his hands myself, I can speak very positively of the efficacy of his methods.

There is one thing about the doctor's treatment which commends itself to me as a Catholic. If I understand aright he is a great believer in counter-irritation; and we Catholics believe in penances for the cure of spiritual maladies. Whatever Dr. Hartt may be in religion, in medicine he is a good Catholic.

This institution will be a wonderful blessing to the poor; yet, sometimes, I think we consider the poor too exclusively, and forget the poor rich men who are languishing in hopeless disease. How readily would they part with their money to regain the blessing of health! But poorer than the sick are those rich men who will give nothing for the relief of suffering humanity. They are affected with a disease of the heart, the opposite of enlargement—a contraction and hardening of that organ; and now we come to them with an opportunity to be cured of their malady by generous contributions to this noble charity.

Let me close as I began, by commending this enterprise as one most beneficent, and imperatively needed, and by invoking upon it the blessing of God.

INDORSEMENT BY THE CITIZENS.

A resolution was then adopted for the appointment of the following committee, with general powers, to take all the necessary steps for the establishment of the proposed institution:

Henry A. Hartt, M. D., 142 East Thirty-fourth Street, New York, *Chairman*.
Rev. Thomas M. Peters, D. D., corner Ninety-ninth Street and Broadway, New York.
Rev. Edward McGlynn, D. D., 142 East Twenty-ninth Street, New York.
E. P. Wheeler, 8 Pine Street, New York.
Uriah Welch, St. Nicholas Hotel, New York.
Stephen de Wolfe, M. D., 138 West Thirty-seventh Street, Now York.
E. H. Davis, M. D., 175 East Eighty-second Street, New York.
Algernon S. Sullivan, 124 West Eleventh Street, New York.
Rev. J. Clement French, D. D., 114 First Place, Brooklyn.
Ranald Macdonald, 33 Second Place, Brooklyn.
Elwood E. Thorne, 133 West Twenty-second Street, New York.
George S. McWatters, 76 Macdougal Street, New York.
Frank J. Ottarson, New York Daily *Times* Office.
C. R. Griggs, Englewood, New Jersey.
George B. Hickok, M. D., 321 East Fourth Street, New York.
Samuel L. Griswold, M. D., 25 West Forty-second Street, New York.
K. R. Taylor, M. D., 257 West Forty-third Street, New York.
John Burke, M. D., 147 Lexington Avenue, New York.
Oscar G. Smith, M. D., 57 West Tenth Street, New York.
W. V. White, M. D., 118 East Eighty-fifth Street, New York.
Edward J. Darken, M. D., 244 East Twenty-third Street, New York.
John D. Townsend, 353 West Thirty-fourth Street, New York.
John Swinton, 124 East Thirty-eighth Street, New York.
B. F. Vosburg, M. D., 257 West Eleventh Street, New York.
James M. Taylor, 1½ Pine Street, New York.
H. Le Baron Hartt, M. D., 225 East Thirty-first Street, New York.

CHAPTER IV.

PROCEEDINGS OF THE COMMITTEE.

The committee thus appointed proceeded to the discharge of the duties imposed upon them with diligence and discretion. They began by organizing a course of lectures and concerts for the furtherance of the project. Afterwards they issued a series of circulars, in one of which there are letters from physicians connected with two of the principal dispensaries of this city, which, in justice to them and to the cause which they have so generously and honorably sought to subserve, I feel it my duty to record in this place.

From E. J. DARKEN, Esq., M. D., *House Physician of the Demilt Dispensary.*

NEW YORK, *April* 27, 1877.

Having an earnest wish that the effort to establish a hospital for chronic diseases may speedily prove a success, it is a pleasure to me to speak in its favor. Being constantly brought into contact with sufferers from such diseases, applicants for "hospital tickets," and seeing how, time after time they leave our existing institutions relieved, to return in a short time when an accession of disease has disabled them, or their pain has become unendurable, and knowing thoroughly how trying to the resources and the patience of the physician as well as of the patient, such diseases as the proposed hospital is intended to remedy are, I feel a hearty interest in its establishment, and a warm respect for the enthusiasm and energy of Dr. Hartt in his philanthropic efforts for the relief of these wretchedly afflicted beings, among the number of whom I myself belong—or I should more properly say *did belong*—for the only entire relief I have had from rheumatism during the last six years I have had through his care and skill; and though still under treatment, I have lately felt the delightful sense of an almost forgotten blessing—the power to move without pain.

NEW YORK, *April* 27, 1878.

After the lapse of another year, during which time I have had an opportunity of seeing the further results of Dr. Hartt's treatment, I cordially attest that the chronic character of my disease is removed.

From OSCAR G. SMITH, Esq., M. D., *Visiting Physician to the Northern Dispensary, cor. of Waverly Place and Christopher Street.*

NEW YORK, *July* 11, 1878.
DR. HENRY A. HARTT.

Dear Sir: It is with great pleasure that I would endorse your proposed plan for a hospital devoted to chronic diseases. It fills a void in our list of charitable institutions, and from your well known success in this class of cases you seem to be the designated person, under the eye of Providence, to establish such an institution for the cure and relief of chronic disease. The patients I have sent to your office with rheumatism and gout, in their severest forms and of many years standing, were thoroughly cured, and are living witnesses of what you can do. I heartily commend your enterprise to all those who wish to do a great good in their day.

Among the lectures delivered for the promotion of the undertaking was one by myself. The substance of it was read as a paper before the Episcopal Church Congress, at Boston, November 17, 1876. As the subject of this lecture is deeply interesting to every good citizen; as the vice of which it treats is a prolific source of chronic diseases; as the remedy which it proposes for the eradication thereof is novel; and as it sets forth my views respecting the physiological character and action, and the medicinal properties and uses of alcohol, I think it proper to insert it in this volume.

THE PREVENTION AND CURABILITY OF DRUNKENNESS.

The crusade against drunkenness during the last fifty years will ever be regarded as one of the most remarkable events in the history of mankind. Originating with a few peasants in a small village in the State of New York, it soon enlisted in its service, on both sides of the Atlantic, immense armies, inspired with an enthusiasm which eclipsed even the fiery zeal of the ancient hermit and his chivalrous followers. New orders of knights and templars arose, which made the earth resound with the clangor of their arms; but, notwithstanding all their daring exploits, the banner of the infidel still flaunts defiantly over the ruin of sacred temples, and the desolation of Christian homes, and just when the world was anxiously expecting a grand assault upon his strongholds, with amazement it beholds them pause to quarrel with their allies, and to discharge their ammunition in thundering and incessant volleys against them. The parties thus furiously assailed have hitherto borne the attack with exemplary forbearance. Profoundly interested in the overthrow of the common enemy, and deeply impressed with the heroism and generous self-sacrifice of these gallant crusaders, they have watched their progress with the most intense solicitude, in the hope that, sooner or later, they would be taught by experience, and learn, by repeated discomfiture and the failure of their plans, to correct their tactics, and adopt the only true, scriptural, and scientific basis of operations.

In every moral war it is necessary, not only to comprehend the nature and dimensions of the evil to be combated, but also, after the manner of the great French commander, to concentrate directly upon it all the battalions and forces that can be brought into the field for its immediate and utter destruction. No time should be wasted in the discussion of questionable issues, and no mistake can be made so certainly fatal to success, as that of associating with the error or the wrong which constitutes the object of attack, a particle of truth or right. We need not go far for an illustration. The conflict which recently shook this country to its foundations was initiated by a body of noble men, who, notwithstanding their uncompromising hostility to slavery, forgot that a crime so foul and monstrous had not and could not have any constitutional rights, and therefore demanded, as a preparatory step, the dissolution of the Union. O! if the untiring energy, the indomitable courage, the enthusiasm of humanity, and the overpowering and immortal eloquence which, for many a weary year, were expended in the cause of that unfortunate combination, had been devoted to the advocacy of emancipation, on the basis of compensation, not with the view of recognizing the "wild and guilty phantasy" that man can hold property in man, but as a measure of conciliation which we were bound in honor and justice to proffer, in consequence of our long complicity with the South in the support of their unhallowed institution, we would not now, perchance, be called to mourn over the ghastly wrecks and ruins of civil war.

The champions of temperance commit a similar error. In their anxiety to destroy the sin of drunkenness, with its melancholy train of evils, they confound essential distinctions, remorselessly trample upon the records of universal experience, misinterpret the judgment of Scripture, and distort the instructions of science. In all times and countries, mankind have exhibited, as a vital part of their organization, a uniform series of ineradicable instincts. No matter into what depths of ignorance they may have fallen, nor how darkly and grievously they may have been tarnished by sin, the belief in God, and in the immortality of the soul, like a divine lamp has shone within them, and revealed their heavenly origin. In like manner, amid all the varieties of position and circumstances, the necessities of their physical nature have asserted themselves in a tone of irresistible authority, and prominent among its claims has ever been the demand for stimulants and restoratives.

It is true that, in the gratification of these instincts, they have oftentimes wandered far from the path of wisdom, and made lamentable mistakes, both in opinion and practice; that they have sometimes imagined that the image of God, by the cunning devices of human art, could be graven upon stone, and have constructed for the Immortal Spirit the most fantastic habitations and associations in a future state; that, in some instances, they have been carried away by the whirlwind of a sensual delirium, so that they have even invested the juice of the grape with the honors of Divinity, and enacted foul orgies at its impious shrine; but, burning still and permanent, though flickering then and dim, hung those precious lights in the temple of their being, which were placed there by him whom they thus profanely insulted, when he wrought out its mysterious chambers in the secret places of the earth. The spiritual instincts, however corrupted or loaded down with multitudinous errors, have ever been considered as powerful evidences in behalf of the sublime truths to which they refer. Why should not the same rule apply with equal force to the physical? Upon what principle shall we reject their testimony, or turn a deaf ear to the lessons of the past? From all the ages we hear a voice, growing louder and louder as it comes, echoing the divine song of the Hebrew psalmist: "He causeth the grass to grow for the cattle, and herb for the service of man, that he may bring forth food out of the earth; and wine that maketh glad the heart of man, and oil to make his face to shine, and bread which strengtheneth man's heart."

It has been laid down by some of the most eminent authorities, that a man who devotes himself to a course of research in any of the higher branches of science should sedulously guard his mind against all bias on the subject of religion, or, in other words, should remain purposely and deliberately without faith and without God in the world. This proposition is totally repugnant to the spirit of a true philosophy. The primary duty and interest of every intelligent being, when he finds himself encircled and bewildered by the mysteries of life, is to institute an earnest and vigorous search for the author of his existence, and, if, haply, there come within his reach a book which purports to furnish him with the knowledge that he is in pursuit of, should he not hail it with eagerness, and make it the subject of a rigid and exhaustive investigation? And if he discover an overwhelming weight of evidence both in the book itself and in the records concerning it, to show that it is a special revelation from the eternal source of life and light, setting forth his being, attributes, and will, and giving a sketch of his mighty works of creation and providence, should he not bind it to his heart with gratitude and joy, and take it with him as the man of his counsel and the guide of his steps in all the ways and walks of his earthly pilgrimage, assured that it can never mislead him, nor conflict with any fact that he may encounter in any department of study? The principle, "If any man will do his will, he shall know of the doctrine," applies not less to the orbs of heaven, the rocks of earth, and the wondrous processes of chemical agencies, than to the higher elements of spiritual truth. With what majesty and power, and almost celestial intelligence, did Newton and Miller pursue their chosen paths, with the Bible in their hands, delighted not only with the resistless manifestations of design which beamed forth from countless combinations, contrivances, and adjustments, but also with the beautiful correspondencies which flashed upon them between the wonderful works and the still more wonderful Word of God! If the leading explorers in our day could catch their spirit and enter the venerable sanctuary of the rocks with reverent head and prayerful heart, they would not become the Quixotes of science, mistaking the fossilized tracks and feathers of birds for links, and "Paradise Lost" for the Bible. They would probably have perceived, ere now, the fallacy of supposing that each of the great periods of creation must have expired before its successor began; for inasmuch as geology discloses that divers species of plants and of animals, both marine and terrestrial, appeared during the enormous range between the commencement of the Silurian and the termination of the Tertiary epochs, they would have inferred that those species were the products of repeated acts of creation, and that the periods which the different classes embrace necessarily overlapped each other. And they would have seen, moreover, that the Mosaic vision determines only the order in which the periods began, and that the revelations of nature entirely agree therewith. You will not wonder, then, that ere I seek to penetrate the arcana of science, and inquire of her oracles, I pause to ascertain if, on the great question before us involving such manifold and momentous interests, the divine storehouse of light and wisdom can afford us any material aid in its elucidation.

It is a significant fact that the first instance in which we observe the mention of wine therein, it appears in all its potency, and lays prostrate in his tent the noble patriarch who had miraculously escaped the deluge. I pass by the imposition practiced upon Lot, and ask you to look with me upon one of the most impressive scenes in history. A majestic personage comes forth with bread and wine to meet the father of the faithful, who gives him tithes of all. In the one hundred and tenth psalm a notable allusion is made to him: "The Lord said unto my Lord, sit thou at my right hand, until I make thine enemies thy footstool. The Lord shall send the rod of thy strength out of Zion: rule thou in the midst of thine enemies. Thy people shall be willing in the day of thy power, in the beauties of holiness from the womb of the morning: thou hast the dew of thy youth. The Lord hath sworn, and will not repent, Thou art a priest forever after the order of Melchizedek." And St. Paul, in his great epistle to the Hebrews, says: "For this Melchizedek, King of Salem, priest of the Most High God, who met Abraham returning from the slaughter of the kings, and blessed him, to whom also Abraham gave a tenth part of all; first being by interpretation King of Righteousness, and after that also King of Salem, which is King of Peace, without father, without mother, without descent, having neither beginning of days, nor end of life; but made like unto the Son of God; abideth a priest continually." Was this he who afterwards appeared in the same likeness walking in the midst of the burning fiery furnace?

In the Hebrew scriptures frequent reference is made to wine as a blessing.

"Thou shalt observe the feast of tabernacles seven days; after that thou hast gathered in thy corn and thy wine; and thou shalt rejoice in thy feast, thou, and thy son, and thy daughter, and thy man servant and thy maid servant, and the Levite, the stranger, the fatherless, and the widow, that are within thy gates." "And it shall come to pass that if ye shall hearken diligently to my commandments which I commanded you this day to love the Lord your God, and to serve him with all your heart and with all your soul, that I will give you the rain of your land in his due season, the first rain, and the latter rain, that thou mayest gather in thy corn, and thy wine, and thine oil."

"But it shall come to pass, if thou wilt not hearken unto the voice of the Lord thy God, to observe to do all his commandments and his statutes which I commanded thee this day: that all these curses shall come upon thee. * * * Thou shalt plant vineyards and dress them, but shalt neither drink of the wine, nor gather the grapes, for the worms shall eat them. * * * The Lord shall bring a nation against thee from far * * * and he shall eat the fruit of thy cattle, and the fruit of thy land, until thou be destroyed; which also shall not leave thee either corn, wine or oil, or the increase of thy kine, or flocks of thy sheep, until he have destroyed thee."

"Wherefore, it shall come to pass, if ye hearken to these judgments, and keep and do them, that the Lord thy God shall keep unto thee the covenant and the mercy which he sware unto thy fathers; and he will love thee, and bless thee, and multiply thee; he will also bless the fruit of thy womb, and the fruit of thy land, thy corn, and thy wine, and thine oil, the increase of thy kine, and the flocks of thy sheep, in the land which he sware unto thy fathers to give thee."

"The Lord hath sworn by his right hand, and by the arm of his strength, surely I will no more give thy corn to be meat for thine enemies; and the sons of the stranger shall not drink thy wine for which thou hast labored; but they that have gathered it shall eat it, and praise the Lord; and they that have brought it together shall drink it in the courts of my holiness."

The combination of wine with flour and oil in their sacrifices requires consideration.

"This is that which thou shalt offer upon the altar: two lambs of the first year, day by day continually. The one lamb thou shalt offer in the morning, and the other lamb thou shalt offer at even; and with the one lamb a tenth deal of flour, mingled with the fourth part of an hin of beaten oil, and the fourth part of an hin of wine for a drink offering; and the other lamb thou shalt offer at even, and shalt do thereto according to the meat offering of the morning, and according to the drink offering thereof, for a sweet savor, an offering made by fire unto the Lord. This shall be a continual burnt offering throughout your generations, at the door of the tabernacle of the congregation before the Lord, where I will meet you to speak there unto thee."

"And ye shall offer when ye wave the sheaf an he lamb, without blemish, of the first year, for a burnt offering unto the Lord. And the meat offering thereof shall be two tenth deals of fine flour, mingled with oil, an offering made by fire unto the Lord for a sweet savor; and the drink offering thereof shall be of wine—the fourth part of an hin."

The character of the wine should be noted.

"In the holy place shalt thou cause the strong wine to be poured unto the Lord, for a drink offering."

But I will not linger in the twilight. The long foretold era arrived, and the light of the world appeared. The Prophet of Nazareth was about to enter upon his illustrious ministry. He attended a marriage festival, and chose as the subject for his first miracle the conversion of water into wine. He went forth among the people a mighty teacher and a genuine man. He came eating and drinking, and the benighted Pharisees cried out: "Behold a gluttonous man and a wine-bibber, a friend of publicans and sinners!" The great tragedy in the annals of time drew near. In an upper chamber he held his last interview with his disciples, and instituted that blessed Sacrament, which will continue as the memorial of his dying love till he shall come again in his glory, and all the holy angels with him; and he selected as one of the elements of that sacred institution, that very juice of the grape, which he had already consecrated at the marriage feast in Cana of Galilee, and said unto them: "This is my blood of the New Testament, which is shed for many for the remission of sins; but I say unto you, I will not drink henceforth of this fruit of the vine until I drink it anew with you in my Father's kingdom." And then, as they were about to go out into the awful shadows of Gethsemane, he added: "I appoint unto you a kingdom as my Father has appointed unto me, that you may eat and drink at my table in my kingdom, and sit on thrones judging the twelve tribes of Israel."

An attempt has been made to destroy the whole force of this argument by the pretence that the wine which was made and approved by Christ, and all that is sanctioned by Scripture, was simply the unfermented juice of the grape. It is inconceivable to me that any man who has thoroughly examined the subject could entertain for a moment such an unwarrantable assumption. The glaring cases of Noah and Lot seem like two great tower bells forever ringing to notify mankind throughout all generations that the wine of

Scripture was a genuine stimulant, and that if taken in immoderate quantities it would act as a narcotic. The unfermented juice of the grape is an insipid beverage, difficult, if not impossible to preserve for any length of time, of no special advantage as an article of food, and utterly worthless for medicinal purposes. It was never in vogue among the Jews, except in connection with some of their ceremonials or fasts, and then as an instrument of penance. It is incredible that its production was the result of the miracle which ushered in the Christian dispensation; and it is obvious from the rebuke administered to the Church of Corinth, that it was not the description of wine appointed to be used in the holy communion: "When ye come together, therefore, into one place, this is not to eat the Lord's supper; for in eating, every one taketh before other his own supper, and one is hungry and another is drunken. What! have ye not houses to eat and to drink in, or despise ye the Church of God, and shame them that have not?" Besides, on the word of a physician, I solemnly declare that it is a libel upon the sagacity of that prince of men, the Apostle Paul, to suppose that he recommended to Timothy this caricature of a medicine "for his stomach's sake and for his often infirmities." If our antagonists sincerely believe in its virtues—if they think that it is preëminently delicious, nutritious, restorative, and in every way desirable to make men healthy and wise, why do they not expend a portion of their energies in an effort to effect its manufacture on a large scale, and its substitution for that which they deem the deadly poison of alcohol?

The questions which have been raised with regard to the philology of the subject are of little importance. It is possible that *tirosh* may admit of a double signification; but there can be no doubt that both *yayin* and *oinos* are used only to denote fermented wine; and they are employed in a sufficient number of cases to determine the point in dispute with absolute certainty.

It has latterly become the fashion in certain circles to denounce alcohol on account of the meanness of its origin. It is, we are told, the offspring of fermentation, and is indebted for its existence to the death of food, and, therefore, it must be reduced to the lowest grade of venomous and detestable poisons. The following emphatic language is taken from a pamphlet issued by the temperance publication house of New York:

"Alcohol is not found in nature. God never created a particle of it. * * * * Having no legitimate use as a drink or remedy, being a poison and a curse, a deadly enemy to health, peace, and human happiness, a special weapon of warfare against morality, virtue, and Christianity, the production, sale or purchase of alcohol, giving it to others, or its use as a beverage in the form of spirituous liquors * * * * is a blasphemous defiance of Almighty God, a war waged for the frustration of his divine purposes and designs, a violation of every one of the ten commandments and of every precept of the Gospel, and it is the blackest and vilest treason against humanity. * * * * Alcoholic spirits, wine, or beer can only be produced by the destruction of food."

O fools, and slow of heart to believe all that the Scriptures have written! Do ye not know that from the gloom, and agony, and ignominy, and death of the cross, life and immortality have sprung to light? "Verily, verily, I say unto you, except a corn of wheat fall into the ground and die, it abideth alone, but if it die, it bringeth forth much fruit." "Thou fool, that which thou sowest is not quickened except it die." It is just this fact, that wine possesses a stimulating and vitalizing force which has come forth from the death of food, which gives it all its prominence and significance in the Bible. It is only thus fitted to become an emblem of that infinite power of beneficence and love and source of spiritual and eternal life, the blood of a crucified Saviour. In a similar allusive sense corn and oil are employed throughout the Scriptures; the one to represent his body—the bread of life, of which, if any man eat, he shall live forever; the other, as shown by the parable of the ten virgins, to denote his grace. In the light of this interpretation, with what interest do we look back upon the whole field of Jewish history! What a halo of splendor encircles the brow of Melchizedek, the King of Peace, as he comes forth with bread and wine to meet the august representative of the system of typical sacrifices and ordinances! How pregnant now with prophecy of future blessedness seems every festival and every offering, with its invariable admixture of corn, and oil, and wine! And when Jesus at length appears at the marriage feast, do not our hearts burn within us as we gaze upon that stupendous miracle in which he presents to the admiring guests a gift which to them is a source of joy and gladness, but to him a symbol of his own dissolution? And as he sits at meat in the houses of Simon and Zaccheus, and in every season of social converse and enjoyment with his followers, while words of wisdom and mercy flow continually from his lips, and he eats and drinks with them freely in token of fellowship, and all rejoice under the influence of his divine magnetism, his soul is absorbed with the magnitude and glory of the work which lies before him, and dwells with profoundest interest upon the decease which he should accomplish at Jerusalem, and upon the sublime and ineffable consequences which throughout the cycles of time and of eternity would proceed therefrom. And when the hour has come, again we behold the King of Peace holding in his hands the bread and wine, which now he gives to the appointed ministers of the new and better covenant, commissioned to go out into all the world and proclaim the glad tidings of salvation through his blood, saying unto them: "As often as ye eat this bread, and drink this cup, ye do show the Lord's death till he come."

The proximity of the powers of good and evil in alcohol is sometimes a source of perplexity. But everywhere, in all the realms of observation and experience, we meet with an equal mystery; in the heavens above, in the earth beneath, and in the waters under the earth; in lightning, in fire, in steam, in the explosive power of gunpowder, dynamite and nitro-glycerine, in common salt, and more than all in water, sparkling, beautiful water; for if alcohol, through its abuse, has slain its thousands, water has slain its ten thousands. Beneath the placid bosoms of lakes and rivers, and in the unfathomed caves of oceans, lie the mouldering bones of myriads who have trusted themselves to its deceitful arms. Even the Gospel itself is a savor of life unto life or of death unto death; and it is written: "He that eateth my flesh, and drinketh my blood, hath eternal life, and I will raise him up at the last day;" and on the other hand, "he that eateth and drinketh unworthily, eateth and drinketh damnation to himself."

I have said that there is an instinct in man which calls for stimulants; and in all the countries of the earth they are provided for him in different forms. I shall continue to confine myself to alcohol because it is the chief excitant which is prostituted by the people of this country, and the Anglo-Saxon race generally, to the odious purpose of intoxication. It is, for the most part, held to be a narcotic, or a stimulant and narcotic; and from its effects upon the brain, when used in excess, it is put down in the order of inebriantia. An able writer in treating of medicines of this kind says: "Taking alcohol as the type, they approach more nearly to stimulants than any other narcotics." According to the same author, narcotics are defined to be " medicines which pass from the blood to the nerves or nerve centres; which act so as first to exalt nervous force and then to depress it; and have also a special action on the intellectual part of the brain." And in his definition of stimulants he says, that they are " medicines which pass to the nerves or nerve centres, and act upon them so as to exalt nervous force in general or in particular."

The fundamental error with regard to this invaluable agent is the habit, which has become almost universal, of restricting attention to its power, when taken in large quantities, in certain conditions of the system, to produce narcotism. But I am prepared to show that this is a power which ought never to have been evoked except for surgical purposes, and that since the introduction of chloroform and ether, as anæsthetics, this necessity has passed away, and that in our classification of medicines it should be struck from the list of narcotics forever. When properly employed, it is a grateful stimulant and restorative to the nervous system, acting upon it, not as a spur to the jaded horse, but rather as oil to the expiring flame, supplying it both with pabulum and force. If a man in a fit of frenzy should choose to pour oil upon his fire for the pleasure of seeing a splendid blaze, till the devouring element should seize upon his house and himself and his family, and all should perish together in one common ruin, would you say that the oil was in fault? A walk for an hour in the fresh morning air, when the flowers are blooming, and the trees are waving, and birds are singing their sweet songs of thanksgiving in the branches, is not more delightful to the mind than refreshing and strengthening to the physical frame; but if a man, wearied of home and friends, should set forth on a wild expedition, and travel day after day over a sandy desert without cessation or rest, would you wonder if, at length, his head should reel and his heart flutter, and he should fall exhausted and paralyzed to rise no more? Or would you burst forth in a tornado of excitement against the evil of exercise, and insist that henceforth every human being should abandon the use of his limbs?

The dread of collapse after the moderate use of alcohol is wholly unfounded. It occurs only as the sequel of narcotism, and is exactly identical with that which follows overtaxation of the nervous system, either by excessive mental or physical exertion. The same remark applies to the charge that its imbibition to-day begets the necessity for a similar indulgence to-morrow, until finally an appetite is created for it which becomes uncontrollable. The habitual use of it in quantities which do not cause giddiness and other symptoms of overstimulation, except in some rare cases of idiosyncrasy, is never attended with any such effect; but it is evident in the nature of things that if it be carried to the extent of producing a temporary paralysis of the whole cerebro-spinal system, depression must ensue as an inevitable consequence, which would necessitate a renewal of the stimulant for relief.

A celebrated physiologist has asked why a man in perfect health should have recourse to stimulants. I am astonished at the question. Where can a man be found who is for any length of time in perfect health? The human organism is constantly undergoing a process of degeneration and repair, and, therefore, is never for two consecutive moments in precisely the same condition. The cares of domestic life, the anxieties of business, the wear and tear of innumerable responsibilities, press upon it every hour, and increase a thousandfold its liability to disturbance. I read a story a short time ago under the title of "Imperfect Instruments." A young man named Geronimo, who assisted his father in the charge of a country parish, had just returned from college with a profound impression that everything in the world ought to go on in unbroken harmony, and resolved that, as far as he was concerned, he would tolerate nothing that was not absolutely right. The first thing in the church that disturbed his mind was the position of a tablet to the memory of his mother, which he was anxious to remove, but he was overruled therein by the prejudices of his father. A festival was appointed to celebrate the birthday of the rector, and

Geronimo was determined that the music on the occasion should surpass all that had ever before been heard in the parish. But his ear was exquisite, and it had been lately annoyed by slight discrepancies in the tones of the organ. The organ-builder could not be procured; so the curate obtained a cone and scale, and on the morning of the day of the approaching festival undertook the task of tuning the instrument himself. He put all the pipes, one by one, in the most perfect tune; but to his astonishment and horror, when he came to strike down the full chords of the key, there burst forth only a clash of discords. When the organ-builder entered into an examination of the difficulty, he pronounced that the "tuning was too perfect by half." "How is that possible?" asked Geronimo. "Because it's an imperfect instrument, sir," answered the organ-builder, "and that being the case, you have to make the best you can of it, and not try to get it perfect, for that is not possible." The physiologist whom I have quoted commits a similar mistake to that of the curate. He seems to imagine that the human system is a perfect instrument, and that it can be maintained in thorough vigor by means of ordinary food and rest. I suppose if he were engaged in the practice of his profession he would aim to keep his patrons, when free from disease, toned up to the highest point. He would direct them to weigh every ounce of food they took into their stomachs, carefully adjusting, in due measure, the nitrogenous, saccharine, and oleaginous substances, and supplying them with all the necessary instruments, would instruct them that they should ascertain every day the exact quantity of carbonic acid that was given off, in a specified time, from the lungs, and the amount of other poisons that was eliminated from the system; and would further prescribe that, if at any hour in the morning or afternoon they should experience symptoms of weariness, they should entirely disregard every claim of business and every interest of humanity, and instantly seek repose on the nearest couch. I fear, however, that the failure in his case would be as striking and mortifying as in that of Geronimo. Mankind will never be persuaded to renounce a restorative so convenient and invigorating as alcohol for any substitute or from any consideration which human ingenuity can devise.

But, although its value in health is great, in disease it displays its supreme power. It is only recently that its enemies have dared to assail it in this quarter; and, I confess, that after all I have seen of its amazing achievements in rescuing those who were ready to perish, I could almost weep at the attempts which are made to blot out the proof on this subject afforded by the experience of ages. If there is one thing conclusively settled in the practice of medicine, it is the efficacy of this remedy in arresting the ravages of typhus and other malignant fevers, and in buoying up the system under the shock of severe wounds and injuries generally, and of copious discharges of blood. Who can imagine the multitudes that have been saved by its influence from the very jaws of death? I have myself the most vivid recollection of many a thrilling scene of breathless anxiety and speechless agony, where the life of the beautiful and the loved hung trembling in the balance, and where, without the loss of a moment, it has come and changed, as with a wand of enchantment, the abode of sorrow and gloom into a paradise of indescribable joy. In these cases large doses are necessary in order to vivify and sustain the sinking energies of the prostrated nerves; and the fact that even in the most delicate organizations, when thus broken down, they do not occasion the slightest symptom of narcotism, incontestably demonstrates that its action is always that of a stimulant, and that it paralyzes only by overstimulation. I have seen, furthermore, in numberless instances, the victims of chronic diseases greatly revived and strengthened by it, even when employed in conjunction with debilitating external applications.

The science of physiological chemistry is confessedly in its infancy. Its disclosures, with regard to alcohol, are meagre and imperfect; but, as far as they go, they tend to establish that from the elements of which it is composed, and the proportions in which they are combined, it occupies the highest place as a combustive material, and that, from its chemical relation to oleaginous substances, it is probable that, like them, it may be applied to the formation of adipose and nervous tissues. It is, I believe, universally admitted, that it causes a retardation of the degeneration of tissue—an effect which we would naturally expect from its antiseptic properties, and the increased power which it supplies to the nerve centres. Its opponents have inferred, from this fact, that it must interfere with the necessary molecular changes, and be a disturber of vital phenomena. But the principle vital phenomenon which is produced by the degeneration of tissue is the generation of animal heat, and if a sufficient amount of this force is furnished by alcohol and other combustive materials, what possible injury can accrue to the system? I attach little importance to the experiments from which the inference has been drawn, that it diminishes the quantity of carbonic acid exhaled from the lungs, because, in most instances, they have been made upon subjects who were more or less in a state of narcotism. Dr. Carpenter, in his essay on alcohol, relies solely, with reference to this point, upon the evidence of Prout and Vierordt. The latter reports that in four experiments the percentage of carbonic acid fell, after from *half to a whole bottle of wine had been taken*, from 4.54 to 4.01. Dr. Prout experimented upon himself, *and took the liquor upon an empty stomach*, the effects of which passed off *with frequent yawnings, and a sensation as if he had just awoke from sleep.* If it could be shown that less carbonic acid is exhaled as the result of moderate doses of alcohol, there would still remain the explanation, long since suggested by Liebig, that the increased formation of water which will occur when it is the combustive material, in consequence of the large proportion of hydrogen it contains, compensates for the diminution in the amount of carbonic acid expired. Upon the subject, however, of the physiological action of alcohol, no man has a right, as yet, to speak with assurance. The late Dr. Anstie, whose laborious and intelligent researches give him a strong claim to confidence, and to whom the distinguished author of the Cantor lectures refers in terms of the highest commendation, says: "It is far safer to rely on the teaching of experience at the bedside, and of the daily practice of large classes of men whose dietetic habits the physician necessarily becomes familiar with, than on the dicta of a science like physiological chemistry, which, notwithstanding its rapid progress of late years, is still in a merely rudimentary condition."

I have thus endeavored to show that alcohol is a gift of God, exalted by him to the first rank among earthly substances, and fitted to subserve the highest and dearest interests of humanity. But in proportion to our appreciation of its importance and worth must be our abhorrence of the depravity and impiety with which it has been perverted from its benevolent design, and made the direful source of unspeakable calamities. It has long been the custom to treat this perversion with unaccountable lenity and indulgence, as if it were the sign of an amiable weakness, or unlucky predisposition transmitted from past generations. It has often been made the subject of guilty merriment, and the sweet strains of music, and the beauties of song have combined to cast a radiance around it to gild its loathsomeness. It is time that this preposterous policy was abandoned. It is time that we tore the mask from this abomination that maketh desolate, and began to regard it as a wilful, unreasonable, and remorseless crime, without palliation and without excuse. How long through our incomprehensible infatuation shall alcohol be permitted to serve as a scapegoat? There is no more cause of complaint against it, as a source of temptation, than there is against the various usages and institutions of society which are pleaded in extenuation for the crimes of theft and murder. Nor should any tears be shed over its abuse on the ground of disease, inasmuch as the infallible remedy of abstinence is always at command for the purposes both of prevention and cure. Nor should any weight whatever be attached to the consideration of hereditary taint. The law which provides that the sins of the fathers shall be visited upon the children is imbedded in the very constitution of our nature, and forms a part of that system of retribution and trial which is designed to expand our highest faculties of faith, and fortitude, and persistence to their fullest development. The divine standard, to which all questions of morality should be referred, gives no countenance whatever to this maudlin sympathy. It makes no allowance for dypsomania or congenital diathesis. With unvarying voice, and in tones of burning indignation, it denounces drunkenness as a crime, and affixes to it the most rigorous penalties.

"If a man have a stubborn and rebellious son, which will not obey the voice of his father, or the voice of his mother, and that, when they have chastened him, will not hearken unto them; then shall his father and his mother lay hold on him, and bring him out unto the elders of his city, and unto the gate of his place, and they shall say unto the elders of his city, this our son is stubborn and rebellious; he will not obey our voice; he is a glutton and a drunkard. And all the men of his city shall stone him with stones that he die."

"Lest there should be amongst you a root that beareth gall and wormwood, and it cometh to pass when he heareth the words of this curse, that he bless himself in his heart, saying, I shall have peace though I walk in the imagination of my heart, to add drunkenness to thirst; the Lord will not spare him, but then the anger of the Lord, and his jealousy shall smoke against that man, and all the curses that are written in this book shall lie upon him, and the Lord shall blot out his name from under heaven."

"Woe unto them that rise up early in the morning, that they may follow strong drink; that continue until night, till wine inflame them; and the harp, and the viol, the tabret, and pipe, and wine are in their feasts; but they regard not the work of the Lord, neither consider the operation of his hands. Therefore my people are gone into captivity, because they have no knowledge; and their honorable men are famished, and their multitude dried up with thirst. Therefore hell hath enlarged herself, and opened her mouth without measure; and their glory, and their multitude, and their pomp, and he that rejoiceth, shall descend into it."

"Woe unto them that are mighty to drink wine, and men of strength to mingle strong drink; which justify the wicked for reward, and take away the righteousness of the righteous from him! Therefore, as the fire devoureth the stubble, and the flame consumeth the chaff, so their root shall be as rottenness, and their blossom shall go up as dust."

"Woe to the crown of pride, to the drunkards of Ephraim, whose glorious beauty is a fading flower, which is on the head of the fat valleys of them that are overcome with wine! Behold, the Lord hath a mighty and strong one which, as a tempest of hail and a destroying storm, as a flood of mighty waters overflowing, shall cast down to the earth with the hand. The crown of pride, the drunkards of Ephraim, shall be trodden under feet; and the glorious beauty which is on the head of the fat valley shall be a fading flower, and as the hasty fruit before the summer, which, when he who looketh upon it seeth, while it is yet in his hand he eateth it up."

"For while they be folden together as thorns, and while they are drunken as drunkards, they shall be devoured as stubble fully dry."

"Take heed to yourselves, lest at any time your hearts

be overcharged with surfeiting and drunkenness, and cares of this life, and so that day come upon you unawares."

"But now I have written unto you not to keep company, if any man that is called a brother be a fornicator, or covetous, or an idolater, or a railer, or a drunkard, or an extortioner, with such an one, no, not to eat. For what have I to do to judge them also that are without? But them that are without, God judgeth."

"Be not deceived; neither fornicators, nor idolaters, nor adulterers, nor effeminate, nor abusers of themselves with mankind, nor thieves, nor covetous, nor drunkards, nor revilers, nor extortioners shall inherit the kingdom of God."

"Now the works of the flesh are manifest, which are these: adultery, fornication, uncleanness, lasciviousness, idolatry, witchcraft, hatred, variance, emulations, wrath, strife, seditions, heresies, envyings, murders, drunkenness, revellings, and such like: of the which I tell you before, as I have also told you in time past, that they which do such things shall not inherit the kingdom of God."

Under the Jewish law, in certain cases, the crime of drunkenness was deemed equivalent to that of murder. The young man who madly broke loose from the restraints, and resisted the endearing influences of home; whom no kindness could win, and no authority control; who sacrificed all the higher faculties of his nature on the altar of criminal pleasure, and luxuriated day and night in the excesses of gluttony and drunkenness—upon the presentation of the indictment and evidence by his father and mother, without any inquiry with reference to their conduct, or the habits of his ancestors, was summarily put to death.

Christianity in its commencement did not directly interfere with the laws or policies of civil government, and, therefore, in its treatment of drunkards restricted itself to their excommunication from the fellowship of the church, and their exclusion from the kingdom of heaven.

In one of the quotations which I have made from the

writings of St. Paul, a specific rule is given for the guidance of the church with respect to drunkards and other wilful offenders, both in the case of those who had a nominal connection with the brotherhood, and of those who had not. In the one case it required a withdrawal from all intercourse; in the other a remission to the judgment of God. There can, of course, be no contradiction in the canons of Scripture, and, therefore, when in another place, the same inspired writer says: "It is good neither to eat meat, nor to drink wine, if thereby my brother is offended or is made weak:" he does not allude to intentional violators of law either in the church or out of it, but merely to those who were young in the faith, and who, just emerging from the darkness of superstition, were not wholly prepared for the light and liberty of the sons of God; whose consciences were only partially enlightened, though, perhaps, exquisitely tender and sensitive; who would be liable to criticise and take offence at certain acts on the part of those who were more advanced than themselves; or, on the other hand, might be induced by their example to do that which in itself was perfectly lawful, but which *through their ignorance* was unlawful to them, and so be brought under the condemnation of their own hearts, and be made weak. For the sake of these earnest seekers after a higher and better life, thus groping their way under immense disadvantages, the apostle to the Gentiles enjoined the duty of personal sacrifice upon those who were wiser and stronger, while laboring to help them up to a full comprehension of the rights and privileges of their spiritual inheritance.

The prominence which is given to drunkenness arises chiefly from the malign influence which it exerts in the production of divers vices and mischiefs. It has been estimated that at least two thirds of the other crimes and of the pauperism which afflict this country flow, like streams of corruption and misery, from this terrible fountain.

If, now, I should be asked to prescribe for the prevention and cure of this evil, in view of all the considerations which I have presented, and the whole history of the subject, I would unhesitatingly say that the first great step in its treatment, without which all else would prove comparatively nugatory and vain, would be the recognition of it as a grievous crime against society, a germinal crime which infolds within itself the promise and potency of innumerable offences and sorrows, and which imperatively demands a severe and an ignominious punishment. I can see no reason why it should not be put into the same category with forgery and theft, and visited with imprisonment in the common penitentiary. Why should the whole nation be subjected to perpetual agitation, their sympathies excited, their property taxed, their lives endangered, and, worse than all, their consciences incessantly besieged by an urgent demand that they should trample under foot a boon of heaven which they find healthful and reviving for themselves, because a body of miserable men do not sufficiently fear God, nor regard man, to keep an animal appetite under proper control? Why should we make such a striking exception in the case of criminals of this description? Why should they be treated solely with argument and persuasion more than others who are not a whit more vicious, and perhaps, not half so dangerous to the interests of the community? It was well enough, I suppose, in the beginning of the war against drunkenness, to try this method. The public mind, indeed, had become so warped in favor of this particular form of wickedness, and had learned to look upon it with such marvellous tenderness, that it may be reasonably doubted whether it would have been possible at that time to secure the acceptance of a coercive policy; and, therefore, the action of those philanthropists who have taken upon themselves the great labor and responsibility of commencing and maintaining the conflict, particularly as they have shared in the common delusion, is not only not blameworthy, but, on the contrary, it eminently claims the gratitude of mankind. Their earnestness, their bravery, and their self-sacrificing benevolence will ever entitle them to praise. It must be admitted, also, that they have accomplished important results; that they have rescued multitudes from the gates of destruction; that they have prevented multitudes more from entering upon a career of vice and misery; that they have awakened the attention of the people to the appalling extent of the evil of drunkenness, and, especially, that by the entire failure of their plans to cope with it in a manner at all commensurate with the necessities of the case, they have prepared the way for the employment of the true, legitimate, and adequate method of deliverance.

The fear of punishment has always exercised great power in the world, and it is almost the only motive which can be brought to bear with effect upon a large majority of that degraded class who have become the subjects of habitual intoxication. The dismal walls of the prison looming up before their stupefied imaginations would have immeasurably more influence upon them than any example, however beautiful, or any entreaty, however persuasive. As a general rule, they are in no mood to receive instruction or admonition, and if, perchance, on some favorable occasion, you may make an impression upon them, it is evanescent as the morning dew. It would be mercy to them, infinite mercy, to lift up before them this awful spectre. A law affixing to the crime of drunkenness the penalty of incarceration for a reasonable term in the common prison with other criminals, faithfully and impartially carried out, would do more in one year in the way of reforming its unhappy victims than all the efforts which have been put forth for that purpose during the last half century.

The efficacy of such a measure in preventing the evil

would be still more magical. Branded as a felony, it would at once lose caste, and be banished from respectable society. The rising generation would be taught from the dawn of life to associate it with all that is shameful, detestable, and horrible, and would instinctively shrink from it as from the bite of a serpent, or from the sting of an adder. And if the authorities who preside over our system of education would provide, as an essential part of the routine in all our schools, that instruction should be given with reference to the laws of hygiene and the mechanism of the human body in a degree sufficient for all practical purposes, so that every child would know what he should eat and what he should drink, I am persuaded that drunkenness would soon retire to the ordinary haunts of debauchery and crime, and cease materially to disturb the public mind.

The common law in relation to this subject has always appeared to me unreasonable and absurd; for, while it allows the crime itself to pass with impunity, it punishes with increased severity any other misdemeanor which may happen to grow out of it, regarding it not only as no mitigation, but, on the contrary, as a decided aggravation of guilt. In other words, it looks with the utmost complacency upon an act which exorcises from the soul all its divine harmony, and fits it for "treason, stratagems, and spoils;" nay, which effaces from that magnificent tablet, the image of God itself, and converts, not unfrequently, the wretched perpetrator into the likeness of a roaring lion, which goeth about seeking whom he may devour; and then, if, in this deplorable condition, without reason, without consciousness, as thoroughly insane and possessed with devils as the demoniac who lived among the tombs, he should commit a second offence, the vials of wrath descend upon him, not merely as though he had been directly responsible therefor, but with greater certainty and fury because he was not. I appeal to the common sense of mankind, and ask if this is not a shameless example of legal charlatanism—a shameless example of the treatment of the symptoms alone, with a complete abnegation of the disease.

The system of license is always an anomaly. If alcohol be a deadly poison, unfit for the use of man in a state of health, then its sale, except for medicinal purposes, should not be sanctioned by the State under any limitations whatever. If, on the contrary, it be, as I have represented it, a pleasant restorative and an accessory food, then every man has an inherent and indefeasible right to sell it, and all discriminating legislation which levies a special tax upon the traffic in it presupposes privilege, and is an infringement of natural rights, and a violation of the sacred charter of liberty and equality upon which this government is based. The impolicy of the measure is almost equal to the wrong; for, as it is well understood that it is protective in its design, it brands the trade as with a hot iron in the very act of establishing it, and creates a political faction composed of men whom it has degraded in their own estimation, who will assuredly combine to uphold a solitary interest, and who will give their united support to any party which promises to render it the most material and efficient aid.

In Great Britain, a society called the United Kingdom Alliance, after a stormy agitation of twenty years, has just succeeded in presenting to Parliament a bill which proposes that two thirds of the ratepayers in any parish shall have the power to prohibit the trade in alcoholic liquors. The Bishop of Manchester, after expressing his entire approval of the measure, and remarking that it would not become a law for an incalculable time, added, that when that event should arrive it would certainly produce a " chronic condition of tumult and anarchy;" and the *British Quarterly Review*, which is decidedly in favor of the disuse of alcohol as a beverage, in commenting on the same subject, says: "The bitterest municipal or parliamentary contests that

England has ever seen would be child's play, compared with the conflict which would rend every parish of any considerable population in the country on the question of adopting the act being raised. We have found it impossible to protect our electoral contests from corruption and drunkenness, even when the publicans have only a secondary interest in them. The demoralization of some constituencies at the last general election, in which the publicans acted as partisans, and not, as their wont has been, merely as the tools of the party which paid them best, was such as to fill some not over squeamish politicians with disgust and alarm. What might we not expect of them at bay, fighting for life? We believe there are few towns in England in which they could not command the means, if they set their hearts on it, of defeating the attempt to prohibit their traffic by a two thirds vote; and the means would be such as would probably in a few weeks do more to promote drunkenness, and the evils which attend it, than would the ordinary incidence of their traffic for as many years."

Thus at the end of twenty years the Alliance finds itself involved in a vast labyrinth of perplexities and difficulties, and with the mournful prospect, unless it shall change its course, that every future step will only aggravate and intensify them more and more. Whatever its numbers, or wealth, or power, or virtue may be, as long as it shall continue to level its guns against the instincts and rights of humanity, it will inevitably fail, and publicans and sinners will rejoice in triumph over it. The system upon which its warfare is based is radically fallacious, and must be abandoned. The time, I trust, is not far distant when both in England and America the irrational policies of license and prohibition will be laid aside forever, and the whole force of moral and legislative artillery will be brought to bear directly and decisively upon the head of the real, audacious, and barbarous foe.

CHAPTER V.

PLAN FOR THE ESTABLISHMENT OF THE INSTITUTE.

Thus far the work of the committee had advanced, although the general depression of commerce, and the inability of many benevolent persons to give largely to any new undertaking, however meritorious and necessary, caused its progress to be slow. They had pursued the usual course of soliciting free contributions, but now it occurred to them that there were peculiarities connected with their enterprise which rendered this method, in the main, as unnecessary as it was disagreeable. At a meeting held for the purpose of considering this point, it was unanimously agreed, after full discussion, and mature deliberation, that, inasmuch as it was designed to employ every variety of bath and other agencies which are used for the preservation of health, as well as for the cure of disease, and some of which are regarded as luxuries, the institution, without relinquishing its charitable feature, could be founded upon the ordinary principles of business. They then drew up and ordered to be printed the statement which follows:

The committee appointed at a meeting of the citizens of New York to take the necessary steps for the establishment of an institution for the treatment and cure of chronic diseases, decided, at a special meeting held October 12, 1877, that the best method for accomplishing this purpose is the formation of a joint stock association, with a capital of five hundred thousand dollars ($500,000), divided into twenty-five thousand shares of twenty dollars ($20) each.

A sufficient amount of the stock of this association will be set aside, to be sold to the friends and promoters of the undertaking, and the funds thus obtained will be devoted to the leasing, purchase, or erection of a suitable building for the objects of the institution in the discretion of the board of directors. The necessary expenses incident to the promotion of this enterprise shall also be paid from said funds.

Each share of the stock will entitle the holder, or his assignee, to the use of the sanitary agencies of the institution, to the full amount paid by the purchaser of the share. The form adopted will be coupons attached to each share of the stock, which coupons at their face value will be received at the institution in payment for its baths, or the use of its other sanitary and medical agencies, at the regular rates.

The name proposed for the institution is the "Columbian Institute for the Preservation of Health and the Cure of Chronic Diseases."

A certain portion of its rooms, board, and medicines, and of the use of all its remedial services, agencies, and appliances shall be given to patients who are unable to pay, for the purpose of effecting their cure; and this department, when once defined, shall never be curtailed, but may from time to time be increased by the vote of the directors: in no case, however, shall any of the benefits of the institution be conferred gratuitously upon patients who can afford to pay; not even upon those, who, from their own resources, or by the aid of their friends, can command the means to make only a very moderate remuneration.

Henry A. Hartt, M. D., shall be the permanent medical superintendent and head of the institution, with the power of appointing his successor; and all the medical officers thereof duly chosen, shall hold their positions by a fixed tenure, and shall not be removable except for a good, just, and sufficient cause.

The remarkable part of this arrangement is that which provides that the holders of the stock shall receive again

PLAN FOR THE ESTABLISHMENT OF THE INSTITUTE. 107

the full amount given by them, in the way of baths, and other agencies, and of medical services, and at the same time shall retain their share or shares as an investment in the institution. As my aim, from the first, has been to establish it on a professional, and not a private foundation, and thus to make it a benefit and blessing to the Faculty, I trust that now, when without any sacrifice they can obtain an interest and ownership in it, they will come forward to its aid in this respect with the same alacrity and unanimity with which, on a former occasion, they gave it their signatures.

The charitable department, I doubt not, will always be an object of commanding interest to the association, and be supplied by them with a generous hand; but, in all probability, it will not be long before it will assume proportions which will demand a separate fund for its support. It would certainly form a fit subject for donations and legacies, and it is reasonable to expect that in this manner it will ultimately be liberally endowed.

A nucleus for such a fund has already been furnished by subscriptions given before the adoption of the new plan, and an opportunity will be afforded at once to those who, from any cause, may decline to become stockholders, to contribute thereto.

CHAPTER VI.

NECESSITY FOR THE INSTITUTE.

It is a lamentable fact, that a number of agencies and methods which are essential in the treatment of chronic diseases have, for a long period, been consigned to the hands of ignorant pretenders and irregular practitioners, until, in the popular mind, they have become identified with quackery. I attended an elderly gentleman, not long ago, who was afflicted with hyperæmia of the brain. In the commencement of his illness he was treated by a homœopathist. After he had been under my charge for some time, I ordered a warm bath for him twice a week. "A warm bath!" he exclaimed, "what next? I have tried homœopathy, and I have tried allopathy; must I now submit to a course of hydropathy?" This anecdote indicates the extent to which the surrender of water has been carried. In the same way, rubbing and passive motion have been set apart as a distinct system of treatment, under the designation of the Swedish movement cure. Electro-magnetism and galvanism were also, until recently, regarded as forces with which the regular practitioner had nothing to do; and we have seen in this city, within a few years, a great commotion excited and fortune made, by a man whose only stock in trade was a simple inhaling apparatus.

The importance of all these instrumentalities has long been perfectly understood by the Faculty, and we now propose to rescue them from the unhallowed hands into which they have fallen, and to place them under true scientific management and control. In accordance with the intimations given at the public meeting, we design that there shall be put into the projected institution every power in the shape of remedy or instrument which modern science gives us; everything, wherever found, or from whatever scarce it springs, which can be pressed into the service for the removal of chronic diseases; that there shall be a separate section for every class of these obstinate maladies that is susceptible of cure, with a physician at its head thoroughly qualified, by study and experience, as well as by original mental and moral constitution, to discharge the duties of his position; that there shall be on the staff an accomplished scientist, who shall devote himself exclusively to the work of investigation; that there shall be a corps of trained attendants, fitted in every respect for the difficult and delicate offices assigned to them; and, finally, that all the peculiar methods and facilities at its command shall be thrown open to the Faculty of New York, for the benefit of their office patients afflicted with these diseases, so that every physician in this city will have it in his power to treat that class of sufferers under his care with efficiency and success; while the plan upon which the institution is founded, if approved and supported by the great body of the fraternity, will secure its management, whoever its governors may be, in their interests forever.

In the memorable conflict for the repeal of the corn laws, in the British Parliament, Sir Robert Peel astonished the world by a change of his views and policy on the subject, almost as complete and radical as the conversion of St. Paul on his way to Damascus. He was placed at the head of the administration because he was recognized as the most powerful champion of the existing legislation, and suddenly he became its inflexible and uncompromising opponent. Disraeli, who was then, as now, an inveterate and unchangeable conservative of the established *régime*, was very severe and caustic in his attacks upon his former ally. He laughed at his pretensions to originality and leadership, and said: "Sir Robert imagines himself a great discoverer, but he has simply found the whigs in bathing and run off with their clothes." But whether the noble knight was a discoverer or not, he certainly performed a great service to his countrymen and to the whole human race. In imitation of this illustrious statesman, we shall endeavor to treat the medical communists of our time as he treated his political opponents. We shall take from them every agency which they have presumptuously divorced from the broad and comprehensive art to which it belongs, and which, through ignorance, they have abused by misapplication, and by their failure to combine with it appropriate internal remedies. We owe it to humanity to break up the system of pretension and chicanery by which health and life are daily tampered with and ruthlessly sacrificed. There is no other department of our social order in which the reign of such barefaced and acknowledged incompetency would be tolerated for a moment. For this startling anomaly, however, the medical profession itself is largely responsible, inasmuch as by some inexplicable fatuity it has neglected remedial methods which it knew to be invaluable, and allowed them to pass unchallenged into the hands of an unscrupulous empiricism. The only hospital in this city which freely and regularly admits all kinds of chronic disease was not, until recently, provided even with a galvanic battery for the benefit of epileptic and paralytic patients. It is supported by taxation, and last year its expenditure amounted to one hundred and thirty-four thousand dollars. According to the testimony of some of its chief medical officers, it does not, as a general rule, aim to cure, but only to relieve the unfortunate sufferers that crowd its capacious wards. Five years ago I was informed by a competent authority that the number of those admitted every month who were afflicted with chronic rheumatism averaged thirty. From a similar authority I have just ascertained that the number has since increased to one hundred and sixty. The little company that hobbled in and then hobbled out again has, by the accession of new recruits, acquired respectable dimensions, and promises, ere long, to become a great army. The general hospitals, for the most part, reject chronic cases; and, when constrained to receive them, they propose no more, except in rare instances, than to afford a temporary amelioration of the symptoms. Their arrangements are made exclusively with a view to the cure of acute diseases. I visited one of them a short time ago, and, in the course of conversation with the house physician, I asked him if the plan of the hospital could not be modified, so that chronic affections could receive the persistent care and skilful treatment that they require. He replied: "It is impossible; we cannot put new wine into old bottles." The dispensaries are equally inefficient. They are entirely destitute of many important facilities, and the chief of the medical staff of the most prominent one in this city assured me that, unless a complete revolution is made in the structure and government of these institutions, the cure of chronic diseases by them must be forever impracticable.

The resumption of the long surrendered and neglected agencies, and their habitual employment in an institution properly organized and sustained by the full confidence of the Faculty, will quickly sweep away all those haunts of quackery which have audaciously usurped them; for it is a libel upon the people to suppose that they would deliberately prefer the application of any important remedy by an uneducated or irregular practitioner if they could obtain it in the best manner under the direction of medical knowledge and skill. The axiom, *Vox populi, vox Dei*, is not restricted to the affairs of civil government. The common sense of mankind can assuredly be relied upon, not less on questions relating to the restoration of health and the preservation of life, than on those which pertain to interests that, however important in themselves, are yet comparatively trivial.

The incredulity which prevails with regard to the curability of chronic diseases must inevitably exercise a disheartening and demoralizing influence upon the mind of every student of medicine. When he sees the victims of these grievous afflictions lying disconsolate and half dead, while the medical priest and Levite pass by on the other side, how must his youthful ardor and enthusiasm be chilled, and how gladly would he hail the establishment of an institution thoroughly equipped with every device which science affords, devoted to their cure — an institution, moreover, which would furnish him with a magnificent theatre for investigation; for here he would have an opportunity, now offered nowhere, to study chronic diseases in every variety, to watch their progress under the most skilful combinations of methods, and to receive clinical instruction from experts in every department.

The advantages which the institution would afford to patients would be absolutely incalculable. Instead of being confined to their homes in despair, or wandering over all the earth in search of various remedial appliances for passing relief, they would find here, under one roof, everything they would require to effect a radical and permanent cure.

And who is able to describe the benefits which it would confer upon the profession to which I belong, and which I so dearly love? Ah! it is painful to think of the batteries that are arrayed against it on every side: the prejudices it has to encounter from generation to generation; the forms of charlatanism ever changing, but all animated by the same spirit of bitter hostility, and casting forth firebrands, arrows, and death! There is not now in the world, I believe, a medicated spring, or bath house, or place devoted to rubbing and passive motion that is not carried on in antagonism to it. Its own weapons have everywhere been stolen and turned against it. Is it not time that we took them back again and wielded them in its defence? The establishment of this institution, under the sanction and by the aid of the Faculty of New York, would evince their determination to save their art from opprobrium, and the successful operation thereof would demonstrate its power to solve the great problems of chronic disease, and thus tend to elevate it to its rightful position in the estimation and confidence of mankind. The solution of these problems would carry with it still greater consequences. Disease in its chronic stage has tested the powers of nature and found them wanting. Its removal, therefore, can only be effected by positive and vigorous treatment. But if a disease can be arrested and cured by positive and vigorous treatment, after it has existed ten or twenty years, would it not have yielded to a similar treatment when it had been going on ten or twenty days? And if many cases of acute disease may, by positive and vigorous treatment, be prevented from assuming a chronic character, may we not reasonably conclude that by the same means many other cases of acute disease may be prevented from proceeding to a fatal termination? Our project, therefore, aspires to nothing less than the explosion forever and utter elimination from the practice of medicine of the principle of expectancy or Micawberism; and its full scope embraces not alone the cure of a large proportion of chronic diseases, but also their prevention, as well as an immense diminution in the rate of mortality.

For this enterprise, then, so vast and beneficent in its aims; so pregnant with blessings to the profession and to humanity, I ask the earnest and cordial support of all my brethren both in this city and throughout the country.

We have it in our power to perform a great work for ourselves and for mankind. We know that multitudes are suffering in despair. Shall we not save them? We know the terrible evils inflicted by quackery. Shall we not avert them?

For this enterprise, I implore, also, the support of all good men; and I invoke upon it the blessing of Almighty God!

www.ingramcontent.com/pod-product-compliance
Lightning Source LLC
Chambersburg PA
CBHW031402160426
43196CB00007B/862